PATIENTS
FIRST

PATIENTS

FIRST

CLOSING THE HEALTH CARE GAP IN CANADA

Dr. Terrence Montague

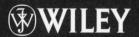

John Wiley & Sons Canada Ltd.

Library and Archives Canada Cataloguing in Publication
Montague, Terrence J., 1945-
  Patients first : closing the health care gap in Canada / Terrence J. Montague.

Includes index.
ISBN 0-470-83511-7

  1. Medical personnel and patient—Canada. 2. Medical care—Canada. I. Title.
  RA449.M66 2004   362.1'0971   C2004-905433-3

Production Credits:
Cover and interior design: Adrian So R.G.D.
Author photo: Julie Hallé
Printer: Tri-Graphic Printing Ltd.

Printed in Canada
10 9 8 7 6 5 4 3 2 1

This book is dedicated to
Patricia Ann, Kathryn Lynn, John Joseph,
Connor Damien, Declan Taylor and
Delaney Kim Montague

And to the memory of
Garner King, MD,
Gold Medallist,
Class of 1964

and

Norman Davies, MD,
Gold Medallist,
Class of 1980

Faculty of Medicine,
The University of Alberta

Contents

Foreword

MARK POZNANSKY, PhD, PRESIDENT, ROBARTS RESEARCH INSTITUTE

Patients matter.

They actually matter most, so the title of Terry Montague's book is really bang on. The system needs to put patients first because they are the whole point of the health care system.

The solutions to our health care problems are not that complicated, and, quite frankly, Terry Montague gets it. He does a terrific job of describing the problem of the care gap and offering the solution: patient health management.

There are two fundamental reasons why readers should take Terry Montague's book seriously. The first is that the care gap represents a huge obstacle to achieving a healthy and therefore productive society. The second is that the gap between the care we need as a society and what is actually delivered is widening in almost every area. We have only to look at the increasing incidence and costs associated with a range of diseases that have large preventable or controllable components: Type 2 diabetes, atherosclerosis, stroke and cardiovascular disease, osteoporosis and smoking-induced lung cancer.

Why is the care gap growing? The reasons seem obvious. The health care system in Canada is being driven by the health care budget and therefore rations the health care dollar. If it were being driven by population health—that is, by putting patients first—things would be better. The struggle, therefore, is between rational patient care and the health care budget.

Patients First offers some fairly specific solutions. As a first step, our health policy leaders have to fully understand the problem and the proposed solution outlined here. The underlying value statement for this entire debate was well put by former U.S. Surgeon-General C. Everett Koop: "That we spend significantly on health care is not the question; that we spend wisely is."

A confounding problem that Terry alludes to is the fact that the future doesn't look any brighter if we simply stay on our present course. Futurists Juan Enriquez (*As the Future Catches You,* 2001) and Christopher Meyer and Stan Davis (*It's Alive: The Coming Convergence of Information, Biology and Business,* 2003) predict changes in our understanding of biology and medicine that will make the explosive changes of the past decade look tame. Powerful new advances in technologies, such as bioinformatics and nanotechnology, will provide previously unimagined opportunities in medicine and in the business of medicine. We will be able to predict and diagnose disease through genomic, proteomic and non-invasive imaging techniques in a manner that we've only dreamed of. Therapies will be much more rational and personalized, and we will be able to follow the specific progression or regression of disease and allow for the more specific modulation of therapy. The opportunities for improved patient health will be enormous. Equally enormous, however, will be the potential costs to the health care system if the developments are not managed properly.

For one thing, proper management means closing the care gap, meaning that a much greater percentage of patients with diseases such as hypertension, osteoporosis and Type 2 diabetes, for example, will have to receive the proper treatment in a timely fashion. To ensure that our health care system can sustain this level of care, we have to make sure that the most effective therapy is given to those in need and that we also refrain from wasting money by using high-tech and expensive medicine inappropriately. Research and well-founded clinical trials must be the norm for introducing all new medical/health care interventions. We can ill afford to use our health care dollars on diagnostic, surgical or medical interventions that have not been proven efficacious.

In returning to the issue of budget-based vs. evidence-based medicine, the obvious question is how a system of patient health management, as proposed by Terry Montague, will affect the budget. The short answer is that we don't know for sure. But surely spending money wisely to build a healthier population is a good thing. Furthermore, with a little luck and good judgement, a healthy population may in fact repay the health care dollar with considerable savings, as healthier people won't incur the chronic costs that can be prevented with better care.

Listen to Terry Montague. He well understands both the problem and the solution, which is to pull out all the stops to put the patients first. He advocates patient health management to close the many care gaps. This will result in improved health for millions of Canadians and then, if we do it right, by emphasizing research and evidence-based health care and not merely budgets, our health care system will become more cost effective and our population healthier and more productive.

Foreword

ROSS TSUYUKI, BSc (PHARM), MSc, PharmD, DIRECTOR, THE EPIDEMIOLOGY COORDINATING AND RESEARCH CENTRE (EPICORE),UNIVERSITY OF ALBERTA

Health care is an important core value of Canadians. While we can be rightly proud of our health care system, it is time for an upgrade.

In *Patients First*, Dr. Montague offers a critical assessment of our health care system and a vision of how to fix it. The difference between this and other "health care reform" books is that he provides his own insight from many health care experiences in Canada, both large and small, and does not not merely postulate theories of health care improvement. *Patients First* offers what can be described as a popular view of health care delivery—the best care for the most people on a timely basis. It offers a broadbrush scope, engaging not only the perspective of a physician or provider of care, but the perspective of the whole health system, never losing sight of the fact that the system exists to serve the patient.

In my view, this book should be read by the following consitutents:

You, the public: The public must become more involved in the health care discussions on the sustainability of Medicare, particularly the relation of its quality, access and costs. The public voice—your voice—can keep us focused on who the health system is designed to serve—patients. *Patients First* will familiarize you with the concept of care gaps, where usual care is not necessarily best care. It will show you how multi-disciplinary teams of all stakeholders, including providers, patients, governments and health policy decision makers can challenge and improve these gaps through affordable, community-based actions.

You, the providers: Health care providers—the doctors, nurses, pharmacists and other professionals charged with delivering most of the medical care in Canada, and their advocacy groups—often get stuck in their own narrow perspectives. In Dr. Montague's broader view of the health delivery system, you will see that care gaps are present in every disease and are preventing patients from achieving the best possible outcomes, and the Canadian society from realizing the best return on our dollars spent. Turf wars and unnecessarily exclusive thinking of the roles of various health care professionals are holding us back from fixing many of these problems using the synergistic power of multi-disciplinary teams. In this book Dr. Montague describes innovative, yet feasible, initiatives that are paving the way to team-based care and improvements in patient outcomes.

You, the health policy makers: Policy makers also tend to take their own narrow perspective, looking at health costs in silos unrelated to the clinical and economic returns that can come with the expenditures on health care. Again, a broader perspective is needed. Appropriate, high-quality care costs money, and the societal benefits may not be directly reaped by one's own specific department, or silo, within the system—but the clinical benefits do accrue for individuals and collected individuals. And the increased productivity of a healthier population, enjoying a higher quality of life, also accrues economic benefits for the society at large. Things get better, starting with the patient. The good news is that it doesn't necessarily mean we need to spend a lot more money, but just spend it more wisely, with more accent on what outcomes it is buying.

Dr. Montague's formula is quite simple: We need to form partnerships and measure the *care* in health care and relate this to patient outcomes. On a regional basis we need to use this information and work *together* to improve the system.

As a mentor, colleague, and friend, Dr. Montague has taught me a lot over the years. This book is a distillation of many of the things he has imparted to me—read it and you, too, will gain some of his experience and vision. Having this insight is important because health care is important, patients matter, and things can be better.

Acknowledgements

No man is an island. Certainly no one who ever wrote a book. I wish to gratefully recognize the consideration and assistance of the many people who contributed to this book.

Above all, I salute the insights, editing skills and unfailing good cheer of John Aylen of Kelly+Aylen. His guidance through the many interfaces and challenges of the publishing arena was invaluable and crucial to any success this work might have.

I greatly appreciate the time taken by many friends and colleagues who listened, read and fed back verbal and written contributions on the ideas and experiences related within this book. These collaborators include Alister MacDonald, who first gave me the idea to write this book; Bonnie Cochrane, Serge Labelle, Jean-Luc Blais, Siobhan Cavanaugh, Gregg Szabo, Bernard Houde, Robert Quesnel, Lori-Jean Manness, Eileen Dorval, Michèle Beaulieu, Elaine Andrews, John Sproule, Scott Wilson, Joanna Nemis-White, Chantal Bourgault and André Marcheterre from Merck Frosst; and from academia and the health community at large, Jean-Pierre Grégoire, Richard Plain, David Johnstone, David Marr, Kenneth Rockwood, Hertzl Gerstein, Pierre-Gerlier Forest, Glennora Dowding, Ross Tsuyuki, Koon Teo, Mark Poznansky, Brenda Zimmerman, Durhane Wong-Reiger, Sister Elizabeth Davis and Albert Schumacher.

I wish to recognize the tremendous administrative and grounding support of my assistant, Julie Hallé, whose unfailing practical sensibility and sensitivity gave the proper direction whenever things seemed uncertain or ambiguous.

And I want to express my appreciation and gratitude to my partner, Laurel Taylor, for her unwavering support, innovative insights and consistent optimism throughout this endeavour.

Lastly, I wish to recognize that any errors of fact or opinion in this work are mine alone.

Terry Montague
Montréal, Québec

Introduction

This book reflects my professional journey as a physician, from the traditional and individual patient orientation of medicine to a broader vision of achieving optimal health outcomes for whole populations at risk. The central thesis of this book is that things can be better. One way to make them better is to translate the same scientific principles that underlie clinical practice decisions to health policy decisions. As I have become more involved with medical care and patient health at the population level, I have tried to remember to do that. In that sense, an alternative title of this book might be *Evolution of Clinician to Politician: The Value of Retaining an Evidence Base*.

In essence, this is a "how-to" book. It explores how a physician's priorities change with time and experience, and how these changes continuously reinforce the notion that health outcomes can be better. It also describes how some relatively simple processes can work within our existing health resources to make things better.

The Physician as Healer

Not everyone agrees on what constitutes a profession or a professional. I began my professional medical practice, seeing patients and trying to diagnose their problems and advise on the best treatments, in the town of Oromocto, New Brunswick, in 1972. My practice then was carried out in a combination of civilian and military settings.

During most weekdays I was the Medical Officer of the Second Battalion, the Royal Canadian Regiment. This was a front-line infantry unit and we spent most of our time training for war. In addition to responsibility for the medical care and public health environment of several hundred soldiers on a continuing basis, I was responsible for the training and administration of about ten highly skilled individuals in our unit's medical section. And I, too, trained for combat.

On weekends and evenings, I often worked on the civilian side of the local general hospital, usually in the emergency room. I also covered for local civilian physicians in their community offices when they went on holiday. In these settings I performed all the usual duties of a community-based general practitioner, including pediatric and obstetric services.

It was, all in all, a rewarding experience. I felt appreciated by my military and civilian colleagues and patients, and I felt I was doing something important by contributing to individual patients' welfare and health.

One particular experience that brought together all these feelings and emotions for me was the occasion of my first delivery of a baby one night when I was the on-duty physician for the civilian hospital. The baby was in the breech, or feet-first, position instead of the more usual position of head down. Because the head is the biggest part of a new baby, the remaining narrower parts usually follow easily.

There I was: new doctor in town, first delivery, and a complicated one at that. How were things going to go? Well, they went well. I had been trained well and had done well in my obstetrics experiences as a student, and I remembered what my professors taught me. And no unforeseen complications arose, fortunately. Mother and baby came through healthy and well.

The new doctor's reputation soared in the community. I enjoyed the thought of having acted very professionally by delivering a healthy baby in difficult circumstances. I valued the gratification of the instant and successful results.

Interestingly, if faced with the same situation today I would not do the same thing. I would try very hard to get the mother and baby quickly to more expert obstetric help. So, if I am still a professional physician now, I am a different kind of professional, or my sense of what is best professional behaviour has changed.

In the late sixties, when I started my medical training, I believe most students applying to and entering medical school saw themselves as future members of a profession that held the concept of the physician as healer as central to their profession. To become a member of the profession and to become a physician-healer involved obtaining the requisite scientific training and clinical skills to competently diagnose a patient's medical problem and to recommend appropriate treatment to improve each patient's health.

For many, this image of the physician as healer was compelling enough to make other competing careers, such as engineer or astronaut, comparatively less attractive. As undergraduate medical training proceeded, the physician-healer concept was reinforced by the very nature of the training, which is predominantly designed to produce a physician who, above all else, can diagnose and treat burdensome human diseases.

With further exposure to a wider variety of medical role models, other values overlaid the physician-healer role: physician-teacher, physician-researcher, physician-administrator and, most recently, physician-writer. However, the model of the physician as clinician and healer dominated throughout undergraduate training, and patients still think of physicians in this way. My sense is that it is still the predominant image that medical students aspire to today and continues to be reinforced by physician professors responsible for both general and specialized training.

3

The Evolution of the Care Gap

During my medical school years, a major topic of discussion was the embryonic development of what Canadians now commonly know as Medicare. From 1970 to 1990, universal access to hospital and physician services became a practical reality in Canada. Medical school admissions grew. People sensed that quality of care was increasing and outcomes were improving. This era might be considered the golden age of Medicare. Certainly, during this time, Medicare entered the Canadian pantheon of values, alongside such concepts as hockey and fair play, woven into the fabric of our country. It remains so.

During the nineties, the cost of care, an important driver in the health system, became an urgent concern. Those responsible for managing health costs saw restricting access to products and services as an easy way to control costs. Thus began what might be called the restructuring era of Medicare.

More recently, restricting access has had the unintended but adverse effect of reducing the quality of health care. The Canadian public now has a widespread perception that the quality of health care has decreased and continues to decline. This has driven several governmental task forces, the Romanow Commission most notable among them, to seek out the underlying problems and make corrective recommendations for Medicare. One common insight from these commissions is the realization that there is no single, simple legislative solution.

Quality, access and costs of health care are inextricably interwoven, and the continuing challenge for Medicare is to achieve improvement in a manner that is both acceptable and affordable to society.

I think it is fair to say that, in the early phase of Medicare, physicians and patients presumed the existence of quality care and optimal outcomes. But they were not often measured.

More recently, in medicine and all the biomedical sciences, the advances in care and outcomes have been driven in no small degree by increasingly robust and relentless measurement. This is particularly true in the development and acceptance of data from randomized controlled trials of drugs and other therapies. These trial measurements have become the benchmark for establishing whether therapies cause more good than harm or have no effect at all.

The ubiquity of randomized clinical trials is a relatively new phenomenon. Scientific proof that patient outcomes are better with one particular therapy as opposed to another only recently became commonplace in many branches of medicine. As a practising heart specialist, I became aware of clinical trials as a practical tool for guiding management of patients with heart attack only in the early eighties. I became a passionate believer in this tool only in the late eighties as a participating investigator in the first randomized trial to prove that a specific medication prolonged the life of patients with heart failure. The causal certainty associated with clinical trial results produces a certain comfort, a kind of moral authority or sense of rightness, for making treatment decisions for individual patients.

In addition to determining whether therapies work, rigorous measurement is also integral to determining why and how medical therapies and practices work, including providing insights into the human behaviour behind medical decision-making.

In this regard, perhaps the greatest epiphany in the journey from individual doctor to population-oriented physician came when I began to understand the extent of care gaps; that is, the difference between what best care should be, as defined by the evidence of clinical trials, and what was actually occurring in the real world. This understanding was enabled by repeated measurement of practice patterns and it drove the desire in me and in others to contribute more significantly to improving upon less-than-optimal care.

As a newly appointed head of a major university cardiology group, it was very disappointing in the early nineties to discover that the drug most commonly prescribed for treating heart attack patients was unproven for that indication. Conversely, proven therapies were being used by less than half of patients. The existence of these real-world care gaps represented, I thought, a missed opportunity. If they could be systematically closed, there would be an enormous improvement in clinical outcomes for whole populations. In turn, as I later came to realize, closing care gaps would almost certainly also drive improvements in the economic health of these same populations, through increased productivity, in addition to health gains such as increased duration and quality of life.

Since that day some sixteen years ago, closing important care gaps in burdensome diseases has been my primary professional focus.

Closing the Care Gap

This book outlines the principles and practices of what may be described as the partnership/measurement brand of health and disease management. Simply put, the health care formula I propose focuses on using our available resources to close care gaps and improve outcomes. It involves optimizing the use of what is already available, particularly the evidence base of proven efficacious medications. In health care, this is coming to be known as patient health management, or PHM, because it reflects the thinking that health is a broader concept than disease, embracing health, losing it and regaining it, all in the span of a person's life. Having the word "patient" in the name serves to remind us of the patient's central importance to all the issues and possible solutions in health care.

In patient health management, broad, community-based sharing of the governance and guidance for managing and implementing projects keeps those projects close to patients' issues and values. Community involvement, ideally, means an environment where patients and their medical, nursing and pharmacy practitioners see the value of everyone's input in making things better. It provides a sense of practical empowerment and another level of moral authority beyond the evidence base. Patient health management fosters the right balance of access, cost and quality. It uses repeated measurement and feedback of practices and outcomes, supplemented by education and reminders, to drive continuous improvements in care and outcomes.

Patient health management works. The largest single project thus far, Improving Cardiovascular Outcomes in Nova Scotia (ICONS), was initiated in 1997. In 2002, because of the positive impact ICONS was having on the cardiovascular health of the population, the project became an operational program of the Department of Health of Nova Scotia. ICONS is a major achievement. It supports optimal care as evidence-based, seamless from hospital to community, and has patient focus as its nucleus.

ICONS and other similar projects can become the model for implementing patient health management on a broader scale. By adopting the partnership/measurement paradigm of health management where the goal is to close care gaps, the Canadian health care system can deliver the best health care to the most people at the best cost.

Things can be better and patient health management is the way.

PART 1

THE THEORY

Chapter 1

HOW WE GOT TO WHERE WE ARE

A Short History of Health Care in Canada

Health care is a continuum, for a person or a nation.

Organized care of ill patients in Canada began in Quebec in the first half of the seventeenth century to support the European settlers, soldiers and indigenous people of the area. Medical care at that time was delivered by religious and laypersons, largely as an act of charity and mercy. For most of the next three centuries, spreading from east to west as the country developed, religious orders continued to support and provide a significant part of the institution-based health care. Even today, religious organizations continue to make significant contributions to providing health care in Canada, although major financial support, administration and governance have increasingly been shared by the provincial governments.

To provide a better perspective of the faith-based focus that has driven so much of Canadian health care, I asked Sister Elizabeth M. Davis, RSM, former CEO of the Health Care Corporation of St. John's and a careful observer of health policy trends in our country, to comment. She writes:

> An approach to health care that understands spirituality as an essential element of healing has a long history in Canada. For centuries, aboriginal healers have been

committed to health care as restoring balance in the lives of individuals and communities. This emphasis on holistic care is manifested in healing circles, sweat lodges, and use of medicinal herbs. After too many years of ignoring the value of such holistic care, governments and health care providers are once again recognizing the importance of this domain of healing in aboriginal communities and in the broader society.

The first formal involvement of faith-based organizations in health care in Canada began in 1639 with the first hospital, the Hôtel-Dieu de Québec, founded by the Augustines Hospitalières. Since that time, Christian and Jewish groups have been actively involved in delivering health care and in influencing the kind of health care system we have in this country. They have founded community and teaching hospitals and homes for chronically ill and aged persons. Names such as St. Clare's Mercy Hospital, the Jewish General Hospital, St. Jude's Anglican Home, St. Martha's Hospital, St. Boniface General Hospital, Caritas Health Group, St. Paul's Hospital, Mount Sinai Hospital, Youville Centre, St. Michael's Hospital, The Bethany Group, Providence Healthcare, Scarborough Grace General, and the Hôtel-Dieu Grace remind us of the scope of faith-based organizations present in every province of Canada.

Faith-based groups have initiated pastoral ministries and chaplaincy services for the ill and the dying in hospitals and homes throughout the health care system. They have been active in the establishment of ethics committees and services and have been resources for the development of statements of mission and values, as well as policy statements with ethical dimensions. They have been involved in the development of innovative community-based programs such as parish nursing. In the community, they have also developed programs and organizations related to the broader social determinants of health (e.g., schools, homes for abused persons, housing projects, rehabilitation centres).

Whether an aboriginal healer or a parish nurse, a Jewish administrator or a Catholic ethicist, a Lutheran trustee or an Anglican volunteer, a Moslem physician or a Salvation Army pastoral minister, members of faith-based traditions are merging the strengths of their religious traditions with the strengths of Canada's public health system. They enliven their work with a commitment to respect for persons, care, compassion, a commitment to equality and collective responsibility, and an advocacy for social justice. Their presence outside and within faith-based organizations continues the work of those who began the first hospitals.

In the health care system of the twenty-first century, faith-based groups have entered new kinds of partnerships to ensure the development of a system more responsive to the changing needs of Canadians. Within regional health authorities, faith-based facilities have found multiple ways to create new and exciting relationships. Some are now managed by the regional authorities; others have signed affiliation agreements; others have developed shared services; still others have contractual relationships with the regions. In these new arrangements, the faith-based organizations continue to be resources for pastoral care, ethics, and the sense of mission. They continue to help articulate the statements of values and ethics. And they continue to provide financial resources to their own institutions and to others often through generous support of health-related foundations.

13

During the present reforms of the health care system and with the expanded understanding of health, faith-based groups have advocated for the creation of a vision that integrates the social determinants of health and recognizes the diversity among Canadians, including inequality of means and situations. They have strongly endorsed the five principles of Medicare and have encouraged a re-balancing of the health care system to be inclusive of health promotion, disease prevention, mental health, spiritual health, and community-based care, with an overall concern for the wide range of social and personal factors that affect the health of persons, families, and communities.

When all are challenged to sustain person-centred and community values in a changing health system, faith-based groups have experienced the importance of advocacy in partnership. Indicative of such advocacy networks are groups such as the Ecumenical Health Care Network, the Catholic Health Association of Canada, the Lutheran Health Care Association of Canada, the Canadian Association for Pastoral Practice and Education, the Denominational Association of British Columbia, and the Christian Health Association of Alberta.

As governments set out to redesign this country's health system, faith-based groups relentlessly remind policy-makers about the place of values: respect for the person, compassion, inclusiveness, caring, equity, social justice, and collective responsibility. They have called the attention of decision-makers to the importance of principles such as the right to health care regardless of wealth or status, the understanding of health care as a service and not a commodity, a relationship between the provider and the patient based on trust, and a commitment to wise stewardship. The opening words of their recently drafted *Health Care Covenant for all People in Canada* challenge all of us to remember these principles and values: "As members of a national community, we in Canada understand that a community actively promotes and nurtures health through compassion, mutuality, care, trust, respect, security and active attention to what justice requires of us. Thus, in fulfillment of our mutual responsibilities, we and our governments solemnly promise to actively pursue and safeguard a holistic and integrated vision of health care for all people in Canada."

A second key step in the evolution of systematized health care came with the creation of a formalized medical service to support the Canadian military during the events of the Northwest Rebellion in 1885. This kind of care has come to be known as case management. The primary goal was not limited to treating the individual and his or her illness or injury. Rather, the goal was extended to minimizing disease and injury as it related to the loss of functional effectiveness of the institution. This care model endures in the modern military and many corporations. It also represents, along with support of Aboriginal and RCMP medical care, a direct federal government presence in health care delivery.

From the viewpoint of most people born or living in Canada since about 1970, the health care we experience has come to be known as Medicare. Its principal characteristics include universality of access to most hospital and physician services, costs shared by federal and provincial governments, no user fees for core services, and governance largely by the provincial ministries of health. This model of organized health care has many adherents now, but such was not always the case. The birth of Medicare was not simple or instantaneous. In this regard, Tommy Douglas, the former premier of Saskatchewan and former leader of the New Democratic Party of Canada, is rightfully given much credit for marshalling the forces that allowed the principles of a universal health system to begin in one province, and spread to the others, introducing the benefits that we still enjoy today.

Implicit in the idea of universal availability of health care in Canada is the principle of equality. Medicare presumes to make all Canadians equal in an institutional arena that is very meaningful to them: their health and how they are cared for. For the core services, conceived and provided similarly across all provinces by Medicare, there is prohibition of any competing or supplemental tier of non-public administered care and service. Theoretically, everybody gets the same core care. The equity inherent in the universality principle of Medicare has real political resonance. It is politically incorrect to foster or favour "two-tier" Medicare and doing so would be tantamount to committing political suicide.

To a patient seeking or receiving physician or hospital care in Canada between 1639 and 1970, it may not have been readily apparent that there was a formalized, focused application of care. During all those centuries, even during the modern era of the mid-twentieth century, care was usually administered and paid for on a per-use basis by patients themselves or by a multitude of third-party insurers. Financial concern, and even the threat of financial catastrophe resulting from the need to pay for health care, was real. Medicare largely removed that significant financial threat, at least for core services. Because of these characteristics and their impact on people's perception of their quality of health care and outcomes, Medicare has become a social icon in Canada. It is part of the fabric of the nation.

The Threat—Is Medicare Sustainable?

Not surprisingly, given how highly Canadians value Medicare, the fear that Medicare may not be sustainable is widely perceived as a threat to our way of life. The threat appears to be real. Several governmental commissions, federal and provincial, have recently verified that reality. How did this situation come about, where an institution so revered by citizens could be at such serious risk of failing?

The answer to this question is not clear, nor are the possible reasons for the concern always easy to explain or accept. We have many varied and visceral interests in health care. The issues and the solutions are intrinsically complex and challenging to order and integrate. Nonetheless, I will attempt to answer the question from the dual perspective of the citizen–patient and the professional provider over the course of the last three decades.

After 1970, Medicare services spread rapidly across Canada. Canadians perceived the value of universal access to core services for which there is no direct charge. Compared to pre-Medicare times, Medicare represented a quantum leap in quality of life. This seems very evident to me. A clinical trial is not necessary to confirm it. Likewise, health professionals, and physicians in particular, found the enhanced ability to treat more patients, supported with reliable payment by government, a seductive combination. Things were better in health care. They also were costing more, but we, as a nation, seemed willing and able to pay.

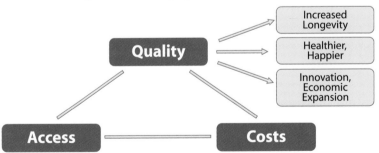

Figure 1.1: The interrelated forces in modern health care are in dynamic tension. As demand rises for increased access to diagnostic and therapeutic services, which drive improved quality of life, costs also rise. To contain costs, downward pressure on access develops, in turn producing decreased quality of care. Adapted, with permission, from Healthcare*Papers* (Montague and Cavanaugh 2004).

Cost is an enormous driver of health care. However, it is only one of three major drivers. The other two are access and quality (see Figure 1.1). They are very much interrelated, as we discovered when we tried to find a model for reconstructing Medicare.

When the necessity for all governments to reduce their deficits or face bankruptcy became evident in the late eighties and early nineties, the health component of each government's budget became a primary target to effect cost containment. In turn, the principal tool employed by many administrators to attain the cost-reduction goals involved restricting access to health care providers and services. And with significantly impaired access came the unintended but absolutely predictable adverse impact on quality.

Physician-related expenditures in 1990, when the reconstruction phase of Medicare began, accounted for about 15 percent of total health costs. Physician numbers were thought to be adequate, or even more than adequate, by many health policy commentators in 1990. There was some sense, however, that physicians were providing more than enough services—and even some unnecessary services. Although very few if any physicians lost their jobs at that time, some actions with longer-term implications were initiated. One was a government directed decrease in medical school enrolment.

A decade after the physician-containment measures, there is a widespread perception among the public and the professional medical organizations of a real shortage of physicians relative to the demand for their services. This is repeatedly reflected in public opinion polls specifically indicating unacceptably long patient waiting times for services and generally increased difficulty in accessing family physicians and out-patient and community specialists.

In 1990, hospital-based expenditures accounted for about 40 percent of all health costs. Hospitals became, consequently, a major health care segment in which to look for cost reductions. In turn, the major budget line item within hospitals—the salaries of employees such as laboratory technicians, dietitians and nurses—became a prime target. Many hospital beds were closed and the level of service decreased. Most significantly, large numbers of nurses lost their jobs.

Nurses are very important providers in our health care system, particularly for hospital-based care. They play a significant intellectual role in mediating and translating physician diagnostic and therapeutic thinking into direct action for the patient. They are the principal monitors of medical care and progress during a patient's hospital stay. Perhaps of equal importance, nurses provide the emotional component for hospitals on a human level; patients perceive them as the primary caregivers. Their caring is visible and tactile. In short, nurses provide the care in hospital care. Reducing their number was associated with reducing emotional care in hospitals, and the diminished quality of care is obvious to anyone who has worked or stayed in a hospital in the last ten years.

Containment of nursing services also had a negative impact on the comfort level and performance of physicians in hospitals. For example, the sense a hospital-based physician has of a patient's well-being at any time is, in no small part, the result of feedback from attending nurses. They see the patients and the patients' families more often than attending physicians do. They are better positioned to place the patient in an integrated medical and social context and communicate this to their physician colleagues. Some of this was lost during restructuring.

There were other negative impacts on physician morale because of the reduction in the number of nurses. It was unsettling to see so many dedicated and effective colleagues separated from their jobs in what, at times, seemed an uncaring managerial environment. In one year, one of my senior nursing colleagues, a truly superior performer, entered and re-entered a formal competition for her position three times.

Also, despite physicians being well positioned to understand the valuable contribution nurses made, there was little formal organized support by physicians to retain nurses in the health system. With time, I suspect there has been a growing recognition that physicians have not done enough. At least I have felt that way and still do.

The impact of all the above produced a widespread sense in the population and among professional providers that value was being withdrawn from the health system and that the quality of care was declining.

Where Are We?

Canadians live in an environment that is associated with some of the best health and quality of life outcomes in the world. We live longer and better than most. Yet we feel things could be better and we fear they may get worse.

There is strong public support for innovation in the health system. There is an emerging impatience with governance limited to elites and with the lack of power wielded by other stakeholders in the system, particularly patients. Within the national framework of our Medicare system, the system really appears to be multiple systems, with primary responsibility assumed by the provinces. The federal presence often seems ambiguous and appears to polarize or entangle matters such as value and funding. Succinctly, we seem to fear for the sustainability of Medicare and sense that the best of our health care system may be lost.

The causes and proposed solutions underlying the tensions in Medicare vary. Perceptions differ depending on one's seat at the health care table. For payers, the sustainability risk is the high cost, or non-affordability. Consumers and providers see lower quality of care and outcomes as the real risk.

Pierre-Gerlier Forest was director of research for the Romanow Commission, which recently assessed the present status and future prospects of the Canadian health care system. Forest takes a broad and holistic view of health and health care; he summarizes the issues as follows:

> Some people think that the long-term sustainability of the public health system is purely an economic issue. Those people are wrong. Even if we Canadians invested all of our country's financial resources in the health system, it would not survive over the long term without a major overhaul that would enable it to meet our needs and expectations. In other words, it would serve no purpose to ensure the economic viability of an outdated system!
>
> The necessary changes must first take into account constant creation of new knowledge, which not only includes new technologies, new treatments and new medications, but also new ways of providing care or of maintaining good health.
>
> Because service organization and professional practices are constantly evolving, new approaches are in fact incorporated all the time into the heath system. But we can do more and better. Useless or obsolete practices present a risk to patients and are intolerable sources of waste to the system overall; they should be eliminated. On the other hand, every effort must be made to spread best practices by promoting the transfer of knowledge from research and clinical innovators.
>
> Recent efforts to review the basket of services insured by our public system failed because they were guided by only short-term financial considerations. Such a review would be worthwhile if it were based on a thorough, systematic examination of the health impact of practices and services (old and new), to ensure that any changes are dealt with proactively rather than reactively.

Another major impact on the health care system will follow from social and demographic changes such as aging, urbanization and immigration.

Let's look first at aging. It, of necessity, leads us to review our approach to organizing health care. At first glance, this means making services available near users and covering, as much as possible, the whole range of front-line needs, including home care. However, a second look reveals that a different approach must be taken altogether. This approach would situate health care in a larger context that deals with all aspects of social policy. The main issue that aging raises is not an increased need for medical care, surgery or medication, but rather our capacity to maintain effective social ties within our communities in a way that does not isolate and, more generally, does not lead to an erosion of mutual responsibility.

In addition to the direct consequences of demographic and social changes, the wide range of needs and expectations must also be considered as they apply to social groups, cultures, generations, location of residence, etc. Canadian society in the 1950s and 1960s was more homogeneous or, perhaps, less likely to question the professional hierarchy or the dominant health care delivery models—our health insurance system was developed in this era and still bears its marks. In the future, we can foresee that the realignment between user demand and service provision is going to become a major factor and bring about a series of changes in how the health care system is administered and governed. The public—users and patients—will make themselves heard in a way they have never done before and demand services that are better adapted and more in line with the needs of a diverse and complex society.

The issue of funding of public health services does not, of course, take a second seat. A system without resources will lose the support of the majority of Canadians. It does not, however, suffice to continually invest more money in the public health insurance system to solve the problems. The system needs to be modernized: what we have learned from at least a decade of experiments is that patients and providers will follow the money, if it is clear that investments are going to be made in support of new and bold ideas.

Managing Health Care: Commitment and Action To Get the Outcomes We Want

Few if any commentators contend we are managing the risks and the opportunities in health care in an optimal and integrated way to attain the best results and avoid unintended, adverse outcomes.

In fact, the concept of "managing" health or disease may sometimes have a pejorative connotation in the Canadian health care environment. It can be associated with negative perceptions when it is seen as a surrogate for reducing "unnecessary costs," or taking the art out of medicine or removing bedside manner from the physician/patient relationship. In part, these negative connotations may derive from cross-border exposure to American experiences with health maintenance organizations (HMO). Certainly, in both for-profit and non-profit models of the American HMOs, business methods and models of management discipline were applied with the goal of fostering both better health and better fiscal outcomes.

However, two things are worth recognizing from the American experiences. First, non-profit American HMOs are very similar in goals and responsibilities to Canadian Ministries of Health—at a high level they seek the best care for their members at the best cost. Second, and perhaps more

23

important, the key ingredient of the business management principles and processes that the HMOs first introduced in a widespread, systematic way was measurement of inputs like costs and utilization of services and outputs like improved survival and decreased hospitalizations (Horn, Sharkey and Gassaway 1996).

It is important to expand our vision of the concepts and processes of management and embrace those, like measurement, that can benefit care and outcomes. We should see the other side of the coin, or the upside potential of management principles, in medical practice. Put simply, applying management principles such as the value of working in teams, the measurement and feedback of prescribing practices and resultant outcomes, and their comparison with existing evidence standards can lead to improved outcomes and cost efficiencies.

One thought I have that might help advance acceptance of management, or business, principles in the health care arena goes as follows. Many modern-day general management principles, particularly the value of measurement as a benchmark and driver, were borrowed and evolved from medical-scientific principles. It is time for us to borrow them back for everybody's benefit.

Accepting, at least for now, that adopting some management processes might be profitable and valuable in contemporary Canadian health care, I think there are essentially two important management questions to address: Can care and outcomes, that is health quality, improve in our present and future fiscal circumstances? If so, how?

Based on all my experience in health care, the answer to the first question is: "Yes, it can improve." And, based particularly on my experiences in health and disease management over the last fifteen years, the answer to the second is: "It can improve through application of the principles and practices of patient health management."

Chapter 2

DEFINING QUALITY OF CARE

Consistently, through time and irrespective of the particular management paradigm, the mantra of people working in health care has been: Things can be better!

While there is a general notion that quality in the health system can be improved, just how quality care and outcomes could be better is not often specified. Only recently have concepts such as comprehensiveness of care, continuity of care, appropriateness of care, or measurement of these aspects of care and their relation to outcomes become practical benchmarks to judge the quality of our health care system.

The Patients' View

Patients must be the focal point in health care, even though we appear sometimes to lose track of that imperative. What serves the patients' interests here? Patients' concepts of quality most often centre on what is visible and what they can relate to previous experiences. For example, a common benchmark in the recent past for many people has to do with their experience in accessing a single family doctor, who repeatedly acted as first responder to all health needs and kept much of the patient's medical and social history in his or her memory. These same patients or their successors may now be experiencing a very different brand of primary care. In particular, there

25

is likely more diversity in how they access medical care and advice. Currently, many patients in many regions of the country cannot become patients of busy community physicians. They do not have a family doctor who provides continuing care, and what physician will remember their care and their health concerns in a shared local environment? Rather, primary care may be obtained at a hospital emergency room or drop-in clinic or by telephone from non-medical staff at a community centre.

It is clear that most people want access to a family doctor, given the choice. One of the most valued gifts I am perceived to be able to deliver for colleagues and friends is not medical advice, but rather facilitated entry for them to a family doctor's practice. This speaks to patients' deeply held conviction that continuity of care is intrinsically related to quality of care. This is one of those issues in health care for which people do not seem to need a large randomized clinical trial in order to draw a firm conclusion between cause and effect. And, as John Aylen, a thoughtful editor, has pointed out to me, this value of patients is also related to personalization of care. In his words: "An institution cannot care. Only a person can care. Personal treatment is important to human beings in all aspects of their lives."

On the other hand, patients may not easily perceive and understand cause and effect when it relates to issues that are not part of their usual health care experience. In this regard, not having direct user fees for health care may contribute to camouflaging the relationship of care, quality and cost in people's minds. Not recognizing the cost of care is not the only risk. It may also prevent people from recognizing the cost of non-care or the cost of not quite the best care on the quality of outcomes.

For example, patients at high risk for heart attacks can significantly reduce their risk by taking drugs that lower their levels of blood cholesterol, a marker of risk. By and large, the lower the cholesterol level, the lower the risk. Several cholesterol-lowering drugs are on the market; some are more efficacious than others. If a patient is diagnosed to be at high risk and is prescribed a proven drug to lower the risk and understands and complies with the therapy, over time the patient may feel that he or she is receiving quality care. If patients realized, however, that there was another therapy associated with even greater risk reduction, which was not prescribed or otherwise available to them, their perception of quality care might change for the worse.

Nor do patients necessarily perceive a quality issue even when they receive no proven therapy for their risk-producing situation. Patients still consistently report receiving high-quality care on an individual basis. Yet even for the most mature of diseases, such as heart attacks, where there is a wealth of proven therapies, large numbers of Canadian patients still do not receive these life-extending therapies during their hospitalizations. The bottom line is this: patients, despite experiencing health care directly, do not always or even often know the potential availability of proven care or how to reliably determine whether they have received it or not.

Is it realistic to expect that physicians have the most up-to-date therapeutic information about each of the multiple diseases that may affect their population of individual patients? No.

How, then, might physicians' working knowledge be facilitated and simultaneously customized for application to individual patient encounters like clinic visits? I think one feasible approach is to involve patients in the knowledge gain and transfer processes. Patients, it strikes me, are uniquely placed to bring not only the best knowledge of themselves to the health table, but also to offer the best opportunity for a visceral accountability of the system that integrates cost and outcomes.

The questions then become: Is it practical for patients to learn enough about quality issues to contribute to their

27

individual care decisions? Beyond that, could patients— armed with better knowledge of the value of treatment options, the cost of these options and the effectiveness of these options in the health system—contribute to how, as a society, we might best balance access, quality and cost to produce the best care for the most people at the best cost?

Based on what I have learned in my clinical experience and from community-oriented disease management projects like those of the Clinical Quality Improvement Network (CQIN) and ICONS networks, I think the answers are yes and yes. And, after recently listening to a compelling public plea for better working knowledge of subjects like health economics for patients and their advocates from Durhane Wong-Reiger, president of the Canadian Advocates Network, I am convinced that patients want better tools. They want them particularly so they can meaningfully contribute to making evidence-based health policy decisions, rather than being relegated to the position of only being able to lobby politicians after policies and laws are passed and regulations established. According to Ms. Wong-Reiger:

> With the evolution of increasingly complex health care options, patients have taken on the role of health care consumers to search for and understand their treatment options in order to participate more effectively with their physician in their health care decisions. Patients are more likely to comply with even the most difficult treatment regimen if they understand the rationale, have participated in the decision and believe it is the best available option.
>
> At a policy level, Canadian patient groups have had to elbow their way to the decision-making table but, once there, have made significant contributions at all levels of health policy. Patients sitting on the HIV Clinical Trials Network, for example, argued the benefit

of comparing new treatments to all usual care rather than placebo control only. In a similar way, arthritis patient groups contributed to drug plan managers' understanding that new medicines not only improved quality of life, but also reduced hospitalizations and time lost from work. Hemophilia, chronic anemia, and other patient groups affected by tainted blood, have fought for access to non-blood-based therapies and these have proved to save costs and lives even as new risks to the nation's blood supply continue to emerge.

Patients are the first to recognize that health care decisions based primarily on saving money inevitably lead to poor quality health care and higher costs. At the same time, patient groups realize the futility of competing with one another politically for limited health care dollars. Achieving better health care for all demands knowledge-based collaboration among groups and with health care policy-makers. However, patients and patient groups need access to information such as health outcomes and health economics data, as well as access to the policy-making bodies, in order to ensure that their input is heard and appreciated.

Broadening the debate to include patients and informing all the debaters are two goals of this book. I hope it will contribute to the enhancement of more evidence-based and more broadly accepted health policy decisions.

The Physicians' View

In my experience, doctors often take it as a given that high-quality health care and outcomes are occurring in their clinical environments. However, this is most often only an assumption. It is not usually based on fact because comprehensive and relational measures of practices and outcomes are not typically built into most medical settings.

29

Although the assumption of quality care may not always be justified, it is understandable in the cultural and institutional context of medical practice. All clinicians, whether they are doctors, nurses or pharmacists, are trying to do a good job. I have never met one who was trying to do a bad job. They are all extremely intelligent, well trained, experienced and motivated by their patients' benefits and best interests. They wish to make the best decisions for each patient and they value very highly any tools or interventions that offer the promise of better care and outcomes for their patients. So, on first consideration, and with all these factors in play, it seems logical that care should be of consistently high quality.

The reality is that quality of care is not perfect; things could be better. Unfortunately, the cultural tendency to assume quality, combined with the absence of an institutional norm for actually measuring quality, may delay or prevent the recognition of gaps in the quality of care.

The upside opportunity here, although it is also a challenge, is to include measurements of practices and outcomes more widely as part of usual care. Reliable measurements offer more than the promise of verifying or refuting assumptions of quality of care: they can also act as powerful motivators to drive improved quality of future care (White 1993).

One topic in the quality debate about which there is little argument is the current shortage of providers. There is an almost universal feeling that Canada has too few doctors, nurses and pharmacists, and that this shortfall has a direct and negative consequence on the quality of care. This perceived threat to the quality of care related to a shortage of people has grown over the last decade, a decade during which the population continued to age and age-related chronic illnesses continued to manifest themselves.

To begin to address this shortage, many medical schools have announced plans to increase enrolment. These moves to improve the supply/demand imbalance in the number of practising doctors will not, unfortunately, have a significant impact until these new physicians graduate and begin to practise medicine. For generalist doctors in community settings, the wait will be about six years; for specialist-trained physicians, the wait for improvement is harder to calculate because it is not simply a matter of adding on an additional five to seven years of specialty training time. This is because of a dichotomy between the announced increase in undergraduate medical school positions and an unchanged number of postgraduate specialty training slots.

The bottom line is, without importing foreign manpower, there may not be a meaningful increase in general or specialist physicians' numbers in Canada for the foreseeable future.

In the context of this book, a very practical problem resulting from the doctor shortage is that overburdened doctors may have great difficulty turning their attention away from immediate clinical problems to focus on innovative tools, like partnership/measurement disease management programs, even though these new tools offer real hope for improved care and outcomes for their patients. In other words, it is difficult to work on improving your business when you are already working hard to survive in your business.

Finally, in the last decade, physicians have been largely relegated to clinical decision making only. They have felt excluded from policy-making decisions in medicine. They sensed or were told that their opinions and values were not wanted, or were discounted by health policy decision makers. At first, some of this negative feedback may even have caused physicians to wonder if the clinical value of their services was being discounted.

For example, a senior hospital administrator told me in the early nineties: "Half of what you are doing in Cardiology is of no value." Initially, I had difficulty understanding the underlying reasons for his statement, inferring as it did a lack of quality from overusing non-proven or non-efficacious therapies. At the time he expressed his opinion, it was widely known from the expanding evidence of clinical trial results that a great deal of cardiac therapy was, in fact, proven therapy. And the evidence of our early practice pattern analyses consistently indicated that underuse of proven therapies, not overuse of non-proven therapies, was very much the larger issue in terms of net appropriateness in prescribing habits. Over time, I came to believe that what he really meant, but did not say, was: "The hospital budget has to be contained and the costs of operating the Coronary Care Unit and the Cardiac Catheterization Laboratory are large. It would be desirable to cut costs in half."

Discounting physician value and input into health policy decision making, which began in earnest in the early nineties, was driven by several factors. The first and perhaps most important factor was the availability for the first time in Canada of a cadre of people formally trained as professionals in health policy and administration. Another was a sense that developed among this new breed of players in the health arena that physicians were untrained in business areas such as accounting or total quality management. The professional health administrators also sensed that physicians might be in a conflict of interest in terms of their own compensation when they made decisions that fostered improved patient access to diagnostic or treatment services. In short, they believed the system would be better off if the business and management decisions of health care were left exclusively to them and the doctors just looked after the doctoring.

Whether they were justified or not, my strong sense is that most physicians felt that having their opinions and experiences excluded or undervalued was detrimental to the quality of patient care and outcomes. In the context of putting patients first, I believe they were right.

Physicians do see their patients and the patients' problems first, and second and third. They buy into the individual patient's risk and benefit options. They work to do the best for that individual patient. This visceral involvement with their patients' problems contributes to a major degree to the stress of medical practice. When they come to a policy table to decide health issues, physicians tend to bring some of this visceral feeling for patients. So, for example, if the discussion turns to balancing patient access and cost accountability (see Figure 1.1 on page 17), physicians may ask themselves: What is in my patients' best interests? Invariably, patients' interests trump costs. This patient-first orientation, in an era dominated by cost-containment goals, may not have been universally embraced by non-physician members at the policy tables. The bottom line here is that physicians take patients' interests personally and they take a personal interest in their patients.

The risk in not having this interest at the policy table, of course, is that the decisions made may not appear good or reasonable to either physicians or patients.

Of one thing I am certain. Based on the evidence, if physicians are provided with the tools, including staffing resources and measurement tools to define gaps in quality of care, things will get better.

Chapter 3

THE CARE GAP AND ITS CAUSES

I cannot remember when my colleagues and I began to use the term "care gap" in daily conversation or educational presentations, but we used it in the literature for the first time in 1997. Since then, its use has become very common. I believe its popularity is because of its utility. It describes, in a very concise and compelling way, a major problem in population health: the existence of large differences between best care and usual care. In terms of improving quality, or how things could be better in our health system, it is not an overstatement to say: "It's all about the care gap!"

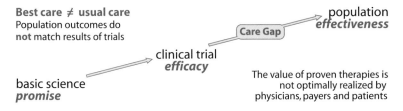

Best care ≠ usual care
Population outcomes do
not match results of trials

Care Gap

population
effectiveness

clinical trial
efficacy

basic science
promise

The value of proven therapies is
not optimally realized by
physicians, payers and patients

Figure 3.1: From bottom left to upper right, this graph outlines the temporal continuum of medical therapy from a promising discovery in basic science, to proof of efficacy in randomized clinical trials, to widespread use in the real world of patients at risk. Care gaps occur when progress is interrupted between definition of best care in clinical trials and the rapid application of this knowledge to whole populations of patients. The primary consequence of the care gap, irrespective of its specific contributing cause or causes, is that patients who could benefit from improved care and lead longer or better lives, don't.

Briefly, the care gap represents the difference between what best care could be, as opposed to what it actually is, in the whole population at risk for any given disease.

In this context, best care is most often defined as therapy that has been proven efficacious, that is better than its absence by virtue of positive results in randomized controlled clinical trials. Actual care, in turn, can be thought of as the level of day-to-day care provided to real-world patients in the community setting. The concept of the care gap and the missed opportunity it represents for patients not getting the benefit from proven therapies is graphically illustrated in Figure 3.1.

Best care arises out of the evidence from basic and clinical sciences, particularly the large randomized controlled clinical trials. In cardiology, my field of clinical endeavour, many such clinical trials have been done in the past twenty-five years to find newer, better therapies for various specific disease states like heart attack, unstable angina and heart failure.

While most new drug therapies are tested individually, they are almost always tested against a control regimen of all previously used therapy. Thus, the clinical trial results give us a sense of how much incremental benefit a new therapy brings to the usual therapeutic package that was available before. On average, the incremental improvement in important patient outcomes, like survival, has traditionally been about 20 percent for most drugs accepted as being efficacious in clinical trial settings (McAlister et al. 1999). This means that a proven efficacious drug, compared to its absence, would offer about a 20 percent improvement in an outcome like survival, over some time frame—such as a week, a year or even multiple years—during which patients were studied in the trial.

As a consequence of these clinical trials, we now know with high certainty that many new interventions and therapies will, compared to their absence, incrementally save lives, decrease hospitalizations and improve the quality of life for patients with serious diseases. The problem, however, is that this knowledge is not translated immediately into action. There are large gaps between what we know to be best care, as defined by the evidence from clinical trials, and what patients are actually receiving.

This is truly unfortunate because, at least for cardiac disease, repeated analyses in real-world community settings show that the use of proven drugs bears out the promise of their clinical trial promise. Their use in the day-to-day community settings, as illustrated in Figure 3.2, is consistently associated with improved chances of survival (McAlister et al. 1999: Mitnitski et al. 2003; Montague 2003, Montague and Cavanaugh 2004; Montague et al. 1995, 1996: Montague et al. for the Clinical Quality Improvement Network [CQIN] Investigators 1995; Tsuyuki et al. 1994).

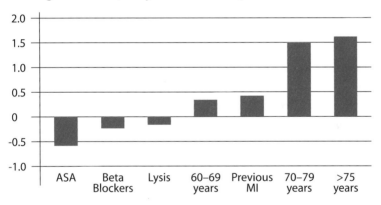

Figure 3.2: Relation of proven efficacious drugs and other important clinical factors to the risk of dying in hospital for 2,070 consecutive patients with heart attacks admitted to four hospitals of the Clinical Quality Improvement Network (CQIN), 1987–1992. In this multivariate analysis, acetylsalicylic acid (ASA) or Aspirin, beta blockers and thrombolytic therapy (Lysis) were significantly associated with decreased relative risk of dying in hospital; previous history of another heart attack or myocardial infarction (MI) and increasing age were associated with increased risk. Adapted, with permission, from *Chest* (Tsuyuki et al. 1994).

One other interesting observation arises out of the comparison between clinical trial efficacy and real-world population effectiveness. The degree of therapeutic benefit or relative risk reduction associated with use of the drugs in the clinical trial settings averaged about 20 percent for almost all of the proven drugs (McAlister et al. 1999). In contrast, in the population setting, the degree of relative benefit associated with the use of the same drugs was often much higher, in the range of 50 to 100 percent, and there was often a greater inter-drug variability in degree of benefit; that is Aspirin, or ASA, seems to confer much more benefit than thrombolysis (see Figure 3.2).

My assumption from these latter findings is that while Aspirin, beta blockers and other proven therapies may have relatively equal degrees of positive impact in clinical trials of heart attack, their positive impact in the population is not equal. In real-world populations of heart attack patients, the benefit of Aspirin is greater than beta blockers, and beta blocker benefit, in turn, is greater than thrombolytic therapy.

I think the reason for this hierarchy of drug benefit in whole populations may be related to their different levels of use in the real-world, community setting. In other words, when therapies are equal or nearly equal in their degree of proven efficacy, their impact in the population is determined by the extent of their use; the more effective therapies are those that are more widely used.

The bottom-line message is that the amount of real-world use is very important to real-world outcomes. As an individual patient or a population of patients, if you don't get the efficacious therapy, you don't get the benefit!

A related message will become evident in the following section and chapters: It also doesn't matter which single cause or combination of causes of the care gap are operating in any individual patient or population setting. If you don't get the efficacious therapy, you don't get the benefit!

The Causes of the Care Gap

The care gap was predicted about twenty years ago by a group of professors in medicine and epidemiology at McMaster University (Tugwell et al. 1985). They looked at the outputs of the great clinical trials of the day. They forecast four main causes of the care gap: (1) suboptimal diagnosis of people who are at risk from a specific disease and for whom available therapies have been proven efficacious; (2) suboptimal prescription of the appropriate therapy; (3) patients' suboptimal compliance with the therapy and/or (4) suboptimal access.

Based on my experience over the last two decades and across many diseases, Dr. Tugwell and his colleagues were very accurate in their predictions. Care gaps exist for all diseases studied and all of the likely causes forecast by Tugwell and his colleagues are contributing in varying degrees to all of them.

Certainly, most health care stakeholders believe there is a care gap. However, opinions on the relative importance of the contributing causes appear to differ according to where one sits at the stakeholders' table. An audience survey of Atlantic Canadian cardiac physicians and nurses a few of years ago suggested that 93 percent felt there was a care gap. Moreover, these health care professionals felt that poor prescription of and poor compliance with medications were the main contributing causes to the care gap (see Figure 3.3).

In contrast, in a similar survey of lay members of the Kiwanis Club of Montreal, respondents unanimously felt that there was a care gap, and that poor access to products and services was the only cause (see Figure 3.4).

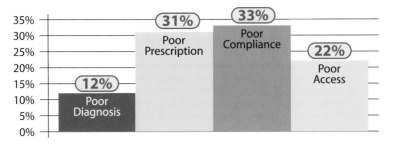

Figure 3.3: Causes of the care gap—physicians' and nurses' opinions of the relative importance of the main contributing factors. Audience survey, Atlantic Cardiovascular Conference, 1999.

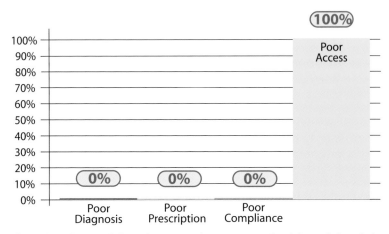

Figure 3.4: Causes of the care gap—patient consumers' opinions of the relative importance of the main contributing factors. Audience survey, Kiwanis Club of Montreal, 2000.

By repeating these informal surveys with many audiences over the years, I have gained two main insights.

The first is that any one person's or group's perspective on the issues and possible solutions in health care is significantly influenced and ultimately determined by which seat they occupy at the debate. It certainly underscores the need for widening the health care debate, bringing more of the players to the debating table and invoking tolerance for consideration of their varying views.

The second observation is that there is a tendency to attribute exclusive ownership of the various causes of the care gap to specific stakeholder groups. For example, patients are traditionally considered to be the main causal contributor to lack of persistence with prescribed medications. Likewise, payers, particularly governments and public institution administrators, are often painted as the group responsible for restricting access, at least in Canada. Shortfalls in diagnosis and prescription, in turn, are most often considered the primary purview of physicians. In short, there is a lot of finger pointing and blame attribution, but rarely do finger pointers look to themselves as possible contributors to care gaps.

My personal opinion is that there is much blame to go around and no one group is exclusively responsible for any one cause of the care gap. Responsibilities overlap and, on the positive side, opportunities to improve things overlap as well. The challenge is to better engage stakeholders in the health debate by more effectively sharing knowledge and working toward agreement on joint goals and processes to make things better.

To foster this enhanced engagement, the following four chapters present in some detail what I consider to be key issues relating to the care gap for which a lot of knowledge and remedial opportunities are available. These dominant problems include three of the major contributing causes of the overall care gap, namely suboptimal prescribing of efficacious therapies (Chapter 4), poor compliance or persistence with prescribed therapies (Chapter 5) and less-than-universal, equitable access to therapies for non-medical reasons like cost or regulatory decisions (Chapter 6).

The other great consistent and persistent issue that merits attention is the significantly larger care gap among older patients, particularly as reflected in prescribing decisions and practices (Chapter 7).

In highlighting the topics of these following four chapters, I do not wish to leave an impression that suboptimal diagnosis of patients at risk—the other cause contributing to gaps in care—is not an issue or target for improvement. Certainly autopsy findings have repeatedly demonstrated that important causes of illness and risk of bad outcomes are often overlooked in clinical care. Less-than-optimal diagnosis of patients is still undoubtedly a significant issue for some diseases, perhaps particularly for diseases that are often silent for long periods from a symptom point of view. Examples of such diseases are high blood pressure and osteoporosis.

In diseases such as these, the patient's first symptom may be a catastrophic complication of the underlying long-standing, but silent, disease processes. For high blood pressure, the first indication might be the chest pain of a heart attack or the paralysis of a stroke. For osteoporosis, the first symptomatic manifestation might be a hip fracture at age eighty-five in an otherwise healthy woman who had unknowingly been losing bone mass for forty years.

As well, in my experience as a heart specialist, I thought that under-recognition, or suboptimal diagnosis, of the heart's pump function was sometimes a contributing cause to patients not receiving early therapy to improve the pump performance and reduce future risk. But, overall, we do not have the same amount of data to characterize the causal contribution of poor diagnosis and make suggestions for improvement that we do for the other principal causes of the care gap. Consequently, my inclination at this time is to leave that cause for the subject of another book and another time.

Chapter 4

THE PRESCRIBING GAP

I first became personally aware of what is now commonly called the care gap in late 1987.

In a conversation with Dr. Richard Crowell, who was chief resident in Cardiology at the Victoria General Hospital in Halifax at that time, I suggested that we might be treating older patients differently than younger patients. As the discussion progressed, Richard and I decided to review the management of heart attack patients at that institution, looking particularly for any age-based differences.

At the beginning, I took what might be considered an intellectual approach to the measurements we were considering. I was thinking largely as a research-oriented person in an academic setting. I wanted to find out if there were indeed gaps against the benchmark evidence of best care in prescription patterns. I did not anticipate how the ubiquity, size and persistence of care gaps would come to disturb, stimulate and drive me as time went on.

My early focus in the field of population health management or disease management was the under-prescription of proven therapies to patients. This is a natural transition for a clinician. It is a reflection of the physician's primary role in diagnosing and treating a patient's medical problems. And poor diagnosis in cardiology, as indicated by the survey results in Figure 3.3, is not considered a big issue by providers. That left prescribing practices as the most likely area to investigate.

Figure 4.1 displays the findings from some of my earliest experiences in measuring care gaps. It represents an example of a care gap in prescription of proven medical therapies among patients admitted to hospital between 1987 and 1992 for heart attacks, still the number one killer disease in the Canadian population (Tsuyuki et al. 1994).

The drugs, acetylsalicylic acid or Aspirin, beta-blockers and thrombolytic therapy are all proven to reduce the risk of dying from a heart attack. So, theoretically, everyone without some strong contraindication, like a known allergy or potentially adverse drug interaction, should receive these therapies.

But, as indicated in Figure 4.1, a decade ago there were large care gaps, with less than half the people, on average, receiving the proven drugs.

As well, within the overall gaps, the gaps were larger for older patients. In other words, younger people were

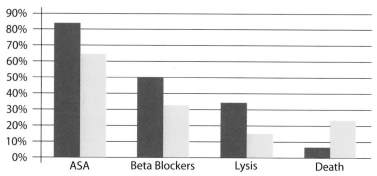

Figure 4.1: Comparison of in-hospital use of acetylsalicylic acid or Aspirin (ASA), beta blockers and thrombolytic or clot-buster (Lysis) therapies, and respective death rates, of 2,070 consecutive patients with heart attacks, 1987–1992. Younger patients (those less than seventy years of age, blue bars) received significantly more of all the efficacious drugs and had a lower risk of dying in hospital compared to the older patients (those seventy years of age and older, yellow bars). The best-case use of any of these proven therapies was about 80 percent of eligible patients receiving the therapy (for ASA in younger patients); the worst-case use was less than 20 percent (for thrombolytic therapy in older patients). Adapted, with permission, from *Chest* (Tsuyuki et al. 1994).

consistently treated better than older people, even though being older is associated with a much higher risk of the ultimate outcome of dying from a heart attack and it could be expected that treating these higher-risk older patients would have a relatively greater benefit.

More recent prescription pattern analyses for heart attack treatment in the ICONS project in Nova Scotia show that, despite improvements, unfortunately, care gaps persist for some proven therapies (see Figure 4.2).

Interestingly, as better prescription patterns have evolved for older medications, the population use of more recently proven therapies is in the same range of use as the older therapies were a decade ago.

In the management of heart attack, optimum therapy in whole populations remains elusive. Things could be better.

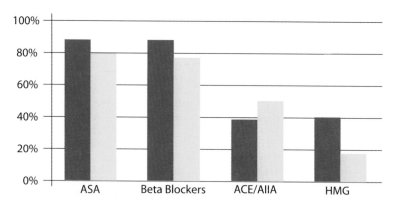

Figure 4.2: Comparison of discharge prescription rates for efficacious drug use among 1,865 patients with heart attacks in Nova Scotia hospitals, 1997–1998. Compared to a decade earlier (see Figure 4.1), the care gaps in the use of antiplatelet (ASA) and beta blocker therapies decreased; for the more recently proven therapies, angiotensin antagonists (ACE/AIIA) and lipid-lowering drugs, or statins (HMG), the care gaps remained very large and similar to those for beta blocker use a decade ago. And there remained a significantly lower level of prescription for all but one of these proven drugs among older patients (seventy-five years of age and older, yellow bars), compared to younger patients (seventy-four years and less, blue bars). Adapted, with permission, from the Improving Cardiovascular Outcomes in Nova Scotia (ICONS) database.

Care gaps in the management of high-risk cardiac patients extend beyond drug use. There are also gaps, or suboptimal prescription, of valuable investigations for assessing level of future risk and in prescription of non-drug therapies for these same high-risk patients (see Figure 4.3).

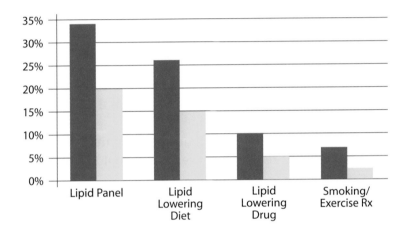

Figure 4.3: Comparison of in-hospital investigations and drug and non-drug therapies among 3,304 consecutive younger (less than seventy years of age, blue bars) and older (seventy years of age and older, yellow bars) patients at high risk for cardiac events in the near future. The specific diagnoses for these patients included exertional angina, unstable angina, heart failure, previous cardiac surgery or angioplasty for re-vascularization and diabetes. The best-case use of appropriate investigation was about 35 percent for measuring the blood levels of cholesterol (lipid panel); that is, the care gap was 65 percent. And, consistently, all interventions were significantly less frequent among older patients. Adapted from *American Journal of Cardiology* (Montague et al. for the Clinical Quality Improvement Network [CQIN] Investigators 1995), with permission from Excerpta Medica Inc.

My best guess is that similar gaps between best and usual management practices exist for all major diseases.

Certainly, our growing experience with asthma, osteoporosis and diseases requiring chronic anti-inflammatory medications, such as osteoarthritis and back pain, confirm a common care gap of under-prescription of proven therapies in high-risk patients with these conditions (see Figure 4.4).

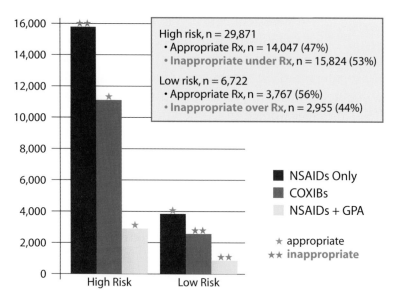

Figure 4.4: Prescribing patterns of chronic anti-inflammatory drug therapy in 36,593 consecutive Manitoba patients, 1999–2000. High-risk patients were defined as older (>65 years) and/or with significant medical conditions such as previous gastrointestinal bleeding, need for anti-coagulants or concomitant therapy with steroid medications. The high-risk patients represented more than 80 percent of all Manitoba patients receiving anti-inflammatory drugs and appropriate anti-inflammatory drugs for them are usually considered to be either newer COXIBs or traditional NSAIDs in combination with gastro-protective agents (GPA) to minimize risk of stomach complications like bleeding. Unfortunately, less than 50 percent of the high-risk patients received these appropriate, evidence-based therapies. Adapted, with permission, from Manitoba Anti-inflammatory Appropriate Utilization Initiative (MAAUI).

Interestingly, among the much smaller low-risk segment of the patient population taking anti-inflammatory drugs, there was also another type of care gap (see Figure 4.4). This was the apparently inappropriate overuse of non-evidence-based therapies in the low-risk patients. However, similar to the cumulative data for cardiac patients, in relative terms of population impact, inappropriate underuse of efficacious therapies in high-risk patients is the much greater potential clinical problem because of the likelihood that people at high risk will die.

The largest persistent care gap in diagnosis and prescription of which I am aware is in the field of osteoporosis. In a multi-year survey and audit in the province of Manitoba, investigators with the Maximizing Osteoporosis Management in Manitoba (MOMM) project have defined the burden of this illness for older women in the population and measured the contemporary patterns of risk assessment and treatment. Preliminary findings from the MOMM study are shown in Figure 4.5 below.

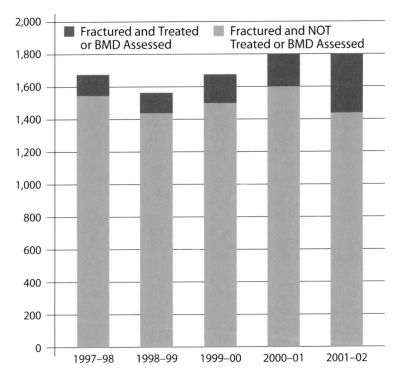

Figure 4.5: Utilization patterns of bone mineral density (BMD) diagnostic investigations or treatment with proven medical therapy for all Manitoba women who suffered hip or spinal fractures between 1997 and 2002. Adapted, with permission, from Maximizing Osteoporosis Management in Manitoba (MOMM). The light blue areas of each bar represent the care gap in diagnosing and treating these high-risk patients. Although care is improving over time, there is still a long way to go to achieve best care in all high-risk patients.

As indicated above, there is a pattern of gradual improvement in diagnostic and prescribing practices between 1997 and 2002, but the care gap between best and usual practice for very high-risk older female patients remains wide. Not shown here, but consistently observed in the MOMM measurements and consistent with earlier results of similar studies of patients with various cardiac diseases, were lower levels of investigation and therapy for women in the oldest, highest-risk patient group, over seventy-five years of age.

In summary, there are many gaps between best prescribing practices and usually observed prescribing patterns for many diseases. How these care gaps are characterized can depend on the stakeholder's viewpoint. For example, payers may focus primarily on what they see as over-prescription of drugs, as in the prescription of risk-reduction therapies to low-risk patients (see Figure 4.4), and refer to this pattern as inappropriate therapy. Physicians may, on the other hand, think of the same pattern as providing an increased safety margin to the same patients.

The bottom-line conclusion, however, based on all the data that I have collected over the last two decades in important chronic diseases such as cardiovascular disease, arthritis and osteoporosis and asthma, is that the great gap, worthy of our closest and persistent attention, is the undertreatment of high-risk patients. If this gap can be closed, we will gain individual and population improvements in health, as well as fiscal outcomes that will have an enormous positive impact on our country's future well-being.

Chapter 5

THE COMPLIANCE, CONCORDANCE AND ADHERENCE GAPS: CHALLENGES AND OPPORTUNITIES

Sir William Osler, the prominent Canadian physician considered by many to be the father of modern medicine, once said: "Man has an inborn craving for medicine."

Despite Osler's assertion of an inborn attraction for drugs, this tendency seems to apply to only about half of the population. An ever-increasing body of data suggests that even for the most important chronic diseases in our society—such as heart disease—half of the patients *discontinued* taking their medicines in the prescribed manner after one year. In fact, most stop after only three to six months of therapy.

Given this fact, an important question becomes: "With such an inborn craving for medicine, why do so many people prematurely stop taking their prescribed therapies?"

Among the four main contributing causes of the care gap—poor diagnosis, poor prescription, poor access and poor compliance with therapy—perhaps the most complex and perplexing is that patients frequently don't adhere to their prescribed therapies. That is, patients often do not take even their first prescription, much less persist in refilling a second or subsequent prescription. This is obviously particularly important for chronic diseases, such as heart disease, which make up the greatest burden of society's illnesses both currently and for the foreseeable future.

One of the problems in dealing with this area is the lack of universally accepted definitions for the specific components of suboptimal adherence. For the purposes of this book, "adherence" is used as an all-embracing term. Other terms can be used to convey more specific features within the broad concept of adherence. For example, "acceptance" means a patient's decision to initially accept the treatment and to obtain the initial prescription and the first refill. "Persistence" refers to the continued renewal of the prescription, in accord with the prescribed treatment duration. "Compliance" refers to patients taking the treatment in accordance with other facets of the prescription, such as correct dosage and timing. Perhaps 80 percent of patients can be expected to exhibit imperfect adherence with regard to their treatment regimen at some time during a course of therapy.

Equally perplexing are the mixed messages and the multitude of terms regarding the compliance/adherence issue. On the one hand, care providers recognize poor adherence with prescribed therapies as an important issue. For example, as indicated in Figure 3.3, physicians and nurses rate poor adherence with therapies as the most important cause of the care gap. In contrast, patients are not necessarily in accord with that view, as indicated in Figure 3.4. And neither patients nor physicians seem to be doing anything in any systematic, concerted way to address the issue, even though it is a big issue. Practically, it seems to be an orphan issue.

From a public health or care gap point of view, regardless of specific terms, the important concept to remember is that there is a missed opportunity inherent in a whole population when patients are failing on a large scale to follow prescribed proven therapy that can improve their health.

From the perspective of economic impact, patients' failure to take the efficacious therapies that have been prescribed for them, the less-than-optimal clinical outcomes that result and the commensurate reduction in productivity in the workplace have been estimated to cost Canada several billions of dollars each year. This is a significant lost opportunity for any society. However, I cannot remember any special or concerted attention given to this enormous health and economic issue at any time in my medical school or specialty training. It may be that the burden and opportunity that poor adherence with proven therapy is creating for our society is now taught in professional schools, including medicine, pharmacy, business or health administration. I hope so, but I am concerned that patient adherence is not receiving the attention it deserves.

I also remain uncertain as to exactly why this cause of care gaps and suboptimal patient outcomes is so neglected. Perhaps it is because no single, revolutionary discovery of cause and solution to the problem is available to capture the attention of health stakeholders: it just isn't sexy. Or perhaps it is due to the difficulty of assigning ownership and primary responsibility for determining causes and suggesting solutions. (These issues are discussed at page 56 in the section titled "Traditional Causes of Patient Non-adherence with Therapy.")

I must admit that I am certainly not without fault in this regard. I was slow to recognize the importance of non-adherence to overall care gaps. For more than ten years I concentrated nearly exclusively on the prescribing gap. I think that my experience probably reflected that of most physicians working in disease management during that same time. Similarly, I am guessing that other groups, such as payers, focused their attention almost exclusively on managing access.

The reality is that none of the four major causes of the care gap occurs in isolation. Multiple stakeholders are involved in creating them and all can contribute to solutions. The underlying causes of patient compliance and potential solutions certainly offer a great case for involving multiple stakeholders working in partnership to close the gap. The larger lesson, though, is that assignment to, or acceptance by,

53

any single group of exclusive responsibility for a particular care gap cause may delay its real appreciation and correction.

Adherence by Disease Setting

The degree of compliance and adherence varies among diseases. For many common chronic diseases, many patients do not persist with their drug treatments beyond six months; the average adherence is about 50 percent at one year for many chronic diseases (see Figure 5.1).

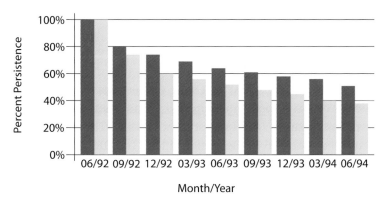

Figure 5.1: Declining persistence patterns over two years with angiotensin converting enzyme inhibitor (blue bars) and lipid-lowering (yellow bars) drugs among 26,000 patients enrolled in an employer-subsidized prescription drug plan. Adapted, with permission, from *Hospital Quarterly* (Sidel, Ryan and Nemis-White 1998).

For some diseases that require drugs such as antibiotics, chemotherapy or anti-arrhythmics, chronic persistence rates may be as low as 20 percent. For situations in which therapy is generally considered life-sustaining, or life-saving, such as following organ transplantation or in AIDS treatment, patient persistence with their prescriptions is much higher, but still not 100 percent; drug holidays are part of the culture, even for some of these patients.

High blood pressure therapy provides a good case study of the compliance gap. It is an important disease burden, both in terms of the number of people affected and the potentially bad clinical impact of having a higher-than-desirable blood pressure for a prolonged period. Management of high blood pressure is the most common reason for patient visits to doctors in the industrialized world, but less than 20 percent of patients have their high blood pressure controlled over the long term (Wahl et al. 2004).

Overall, although there are differences among specific anti-hypertensive medications in degree of compliance, the best-case scenario is a long-term adherence rate of slightly more than 60 percent (Wahl et al. 2004). And, as indicated above, similar persistence rates are seen in many other diseases, including diabetes, AIDS, asthma and following heart attacks (Wahl et al. 2004).

My own personal experiences support these data. Both of my parents had high blood pressure, and it was certainly the most frequent reason for their visits to their doctor. Both received prescription drug therapy to control their blood pressure and both persisted with their prescriptions for many years, although I believe their adherence was less than perfect. In retrospect, I think my parents were like many patients. They probably had some varying combination of incomplete understanding of the risk of high blood pressure as a disease without symptoms and the importance of controlling their blood pressure level, a reluctance to take any medication (possibly because of perceived side effects) or a clash with other life imperatives that led to their not always taking medicine as directed.

The bottom line, though, was that their blood pressure was never optimally and continuously controlled, and this very likely contributed to their premature deaths.

What Is the Gold Standard?

The benchmark for patient adherence with prescribed drug therapy comes from the results commonly reported for patients participating in randomized clinical trials.

For example, in the Simvastatin/Enalapril Coronary Atherosclerosis Trial (SCAT), both an angiotensin-converting enzyme (ACE) inhibitor and a lipid-lowering drug had measured patient persistence greater than 90 percent over almost five years (see Figure 5.2; Teo, Burton, Buller et al. 2000). The drugs used in this clinical trial, conducted at several sites in Canada, were the same ones shown in Figure 5.1, which shows their use in a non-trial, real-world population where their persistence fell to 50 percent or less in one to two years.

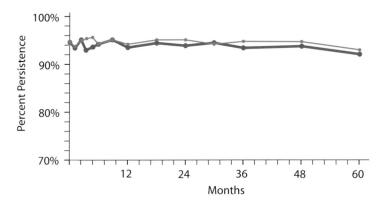

Figure 5.2: Consistent persistence patterns among several hundred high-risk cardiac patients with two drugs—an angiotensin-converting enzyme inhibitor (blue line) and a placebo control drug (red line)—in a randomized clinical trial testing the value of medication in reducing progression of atherosclerosis in the arteries of patients' hearts over five years. Adapted, with permission, from *Circulation* (Teo, Burton, Buller et al. 2000).

Traditional Causes of Patient Non-adherence with Therapy

One obvious observation from the comparison of the utilization data of the same drugs in Figures 5.1 and 5.2 is that the clinical setting and its associated practices and processes have an important influence on patients' willingness and actions to comply with prescribed therapy. Patients' persistence with drug therapy is not just related to drug-specific factors. Other factors in the care environment and its interactions are important as well. The contributing causes of poor patient adherence with medications or other prescribed therapies are numerous.

Interestingly, demographic characteristics of patients— including ethnicity, sex, age and socioeconomic status—seem to play only minor and inconsistent roles. More important factors include patients' sense of the severity of their illness and the complexity of treatment; its costs and side effects; availability of patient social support and sense of self-efficacy and knowledge of the disease and treatment alternatives; and the patient's usual life routine and its likely degree of disruption by any therapy (Wahl et al. 2004). Interestingly, and contrary to previous popular assumptions, it has recently been reported by Schalansky and Levy that the number of drugs taken by patients is inversely related to persistence (Schalansky and Levy 2002). In their study of patients taking lipid-lowering and angiotensin-converting enzyme inhibitor drugs, patients taking fewer medications overall had lower adherence rates than patients taking more drugs.

Theoretically, some of the factors influencing patients' decisions on adherence may be explained by the health belief model (Rosenstock 1974). Briefly, this theory suggests that patients' perception of their own risk/benefit situation or particular set of circumstances is very important to their decision making in terms of persistence and adherence to prescribed therapy. Patients would likely take persistent action to avoid the consequences of a disease with at least moderate severity when they believed that there was personal risk and that taking a particular action would be beneficial and not associated with off-setting barriers such as cost or inconvenience. The theory also suggests that an individual patient may still require some specific stimulating trigger to actually become persistent, even if all the above conditions are present (Wahl et al. 2004).

The relationship between the patient as recipient and the prescribing professional as provider in the diagnostic and therapeutic covenant also has a strong impact on patient persistence patterns. Potential problems in this crucial relationship include the patient and doctor having differing perceptions of the health problem and gaps between the expectations of the patient and those of the physician with regard to risk and likely benefits of therapy (Wahl et al. 2004). In other words, if the physician cannot communicate the urgency of taking the medication and the high risk involved in not taking the medication, the patient is less likely to comply with the prescription.

In general, I believe there is a direct correlation between the quality of patient–practitioner communication and patient satisfaction with care. Effective communication can be a source of patient motivation, support and reassurance, as well as providing a doctor with a better understanding of the influences on the patient, particularly those that might lead a patient to deviate from the ideal treatment schedule (Wahl et al. 2004).

Research suggests that patients want a more active role in their medical care and more information from their physicians (Wahl et al. 2004). Increased perception of patient input into and shared control of their care has been demonstrated to be positively correlated to patients' physiological measures of health and self-reported health status (Wahl et al. 2004). Experiences within the diagnostics/therapeutic covenant that reinforce patients' satisfaction, self-confidence, motivation and positive view of their health status may positively affect their health outcomes (Wahl et al. 2004). Specifically, patients' satisfaction with the relationship may, in turn, play a major role in their decisions to ultimately accept and/or persist with prescribed therapy. In other words, the more patients are involved with their health care, the better they feel and the more positive they feel about the quality of their care.

However, the traditional view of the doctor–patient relationship might be described as being mostly one way. The doctor weighs the balance of a diagnosis with its available therapies in terms of risk and benefit, and then makes a largely unilateral decision. The doctor then informs the patient of the decision and assumes the patient has the understanding, consent and will to persistently follow the therapeutic recommendation.

Various stakeholders in the health care system have objected to this traditional model of provider–patient interaction as inequitable because it fosters or camouflages discord between provider and patient in terms of how each perceives the balance of risk-benefit evidence in making a treatment decision. Furthermore, the traditional model has obviously not been effective in encouraging compliance.

The Concordance Model for Patient–Physician Interaction

Recognizing the opportunity to improve the provider–patient relationship has led to the development of a new basis for this important health care relationship, particularly in terms of patient persistence with therapy. This new perspective on the provider–patient interaction on therapy is frequently called the concordance model (Marinker 1997).

In the concordance model, the clinical encounter is characterized as:

> . . . two sets of contrasted but equally cogent health beliefs—that of the patient and that of the doctor. The task of the patient is to convey his or her health beliefs to the doctor; and of the doctor, to enable this to happen. The task of the doctor or other prescriber is to convey his or her (professionally informed) health beliefs to the patient; and of the patient, to entertain these. The intention is to assist the patient to make as informed a choice as possible about the diagnosis and

treatment, about benefit and risk and to take full part in a therapeutic alliance. Although reciprocal, this is an alliance in which the most important determinations are agreed to be those made by the patient. (Marinker 1997)

Concordance puts the patient first and at the centre of his or her health care.

It seems obvious that poor concordance of physician and patient in the provider–receiver interaction would undermine the patient's persistence with therapy. Fortunately, there is an increasing shift toward improved provider–patient communication and concordance in interpretation of the specific risks and benefits of an individual's disease and proposed therapy. This continuing evolution in doctor-patient relationships offers hope for future improvement in patient persistence and ultimate health outcomes (Butler, Rollnick and Stott 1996).

To illustrate the concept and value of concordance in the physician–patient relation, I offer the following story. This story was related to me by a close colleague whose spouse had been prescribed a lipid-lowering drug to treat her high cholesterol level. The patient, my colleague's wife, initially and steadfastly refused to fill even a first prescription for the medication even though there was overwhelming evidence that taking it would reduce her future risk of dying or having a stroke or heart attack.

This state of affairs was very frustrating for my colleague because he knew and accepted the benefit of the prescribed therapy in general, and for his wife's circumstances in particular. Moreover, he was frustrated by her persistent refusal despite his equally persistent statement of the benefits of taking the prescribed therapy and the risky implications of not taking it. The risks he outlined included much more than the usual clinical statements about decreasing risk of heart attack. It was phrased in terms such as "losing her quality of life" and "not being there for the kids." All in all, it was a pretty powerful proposal that my colleague presented.

When, despite his evidence-based and visceral approach, he realized that he was not getting through to his wife, at least in terms of changing her mind, he finally asked the $64,000 question: "What is preventing you from taking this medication?" She replied that the prospect of taking the drug for the rest of her life "made her feel old and that she felt she was too young to feel old."

So, finally, the real driving issue in the patient's non-compliance surfaced. As my friend puts it: "The beauty of the concordance model is its efficiency in eliminating false assumptions on what motivates patients to comply with their medications." He went on to tell me the real lesson for him was that you cannot generalize when you are dealing with a unique individual. Had he or his wife's physician been an active listener in the first place, he would have been able to identify the issue from the start and been in a better position to deal with it. In the absence of a dialogue, the prescribing physician assumed that he had done his job and believed that the prescription was filled.

In the end, the patient changed physicians and found one who was more open and willing to listen to her concerns.

Who Owns the Adherence/Compliance Issue and What Can Be Done To Improve Things?

Briefly, the answers are, respectively, everybody and a lot.

For a long time, I and many other physician providers had the sense that poor compliance, with its causes and effects, had everything to do with the patient. However, as indicated earlier, if one buys into the concordance model, it is obvious that physicians and other health providers can likely contribute to significantly improved patient persistence with therapy if they contribute to better concordance in the physician–patient discussions of the risks and benefits relating to a disease and its treatment. That is, education of and communication between provider and patient are implicated in resolving the problem of poor compliance with therapy. It is not just a patient issue.

What Works?

On reviewing the literature of what has been found to improve patient compliance beyond optimizing communication, several other interventions have been found to be efficacious. They include education, measurement and feedback, reminders and financial incentives. All have been shown to significantly increase persistence with therapy (Wahl et al. 2004). This is true when these interventions are applied at any one of the patient, physician or pharmacist levels, or at all levels of the care interaction (Wahl et al. 2004).

The Merck Frosst Patient Health team has been actively working in the compliance area for several years, most frequently in partnership with pharmacies and pharmacists.

The major efforts have been concentrated on patient education relating to the patient's disease, its risks and benefits of treatment and the value of persistence with treatment. Patients are enrolled at their pharmacy when they bring their first prescription for the medication. The pharmacist explains the goals of the program and obtains understanding consent from the patient. The patient then receives serial educational interventions and reminders at regular intervals, usually over the course of six months. This time frame is very important because it corresponds to the moments when there is the highest risk for patients to become non-compliant and cease taking their prescribed medications (see Figure 5.1).

Currently the interventions have largely consisted of brochures and video tools and reminders delivered by a third-party supplier. A representative example of the impact of such a patient education program on improving persistence with prescribed medications is illustrated in Figure 5.3. Note that while the educational intervention has a positive effect in increasing persistence compared to usual practice without the intervention, the impact is not totally effective. Declining persistence still occurs, indicating a need for continuous and perhaps more innovative interventions.

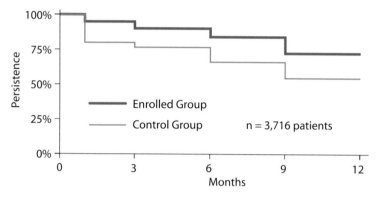

Figure 5.3: Impact of patient education on persistence with prescribed angiotensin-converting enzyme inhibitor medications. Patients enrolled in the education intervention group, represented by the blue line, had significantly higher persistence with their therapy than the control group of patients who received no intervention. On average, the patients receiving the education intervention took the prescribed medication for fifty-one days more than the control group over the twelve-month study period. Adapted from the Merck Frosst pro-adherence program data, 2002.

Based on our own experiences and what we have learned from reviewing others' experiences (Wahl et al. 2004), we believe that the quality of the patient–provider relationship is also of critical importance in improving patient persistence with medication therapy. With enhanced listening and judicious questioning, we think that care providers, particularly doctors and pharmacists, can identify some of the factors underlying non-compliance or non-adherence and target mutually agreed-upon solutions with the patients. Ideally, pro-compliance programs should involve multiple stakeholders in education, communication and repeated measurement and feedback loops that display the continuing results of the interventions to all stakeholders (Wahl et al. 2004).

However, patients should be first in consideration. By putting patients first, as they are in the concordance model of adherence, patients take on a sense of responsibility. They recognize that they are valuable partners in obtaining their own best health outcomes. Then they will act to make important contributions to ensure the success of their treatment.

Patient education should be a central intervention. It should include education about the issues of compliance as they affect individuals and society. It should communicate the preference of the patient–provider relationship as a bilateral one, as well as traditional information on disease physiology and therapeutic efficacy. And, borrowing from our experience with clinical trials, it would be beneficial for improved adherence if patients were informed of and involved in regularly measuring their own adherence and persistence in the management of their disease.

Lastly, I think pro-compliance or persistence programs should also be designed for long-term sustainability, given the nature of chronic illness, even though early focus on newly diagnosed patients may be the most effective way to begin since they have the greatest rates of declining persistence. Using interventions that are affordable and layered in—that is, they become a facile part of the patients' and providers' daily processes, as opposed to burdensome add-ons—would facilitate buy-in from all parties and enhance the effectiveness of the interventions over prolonged periods.

All of this evidence and thought lead me to conclude that everyone in health care should take some responsibility for poor compliance in the care gap. It is truly a public health issue. Any person or health care segment who can foster education, reminders, and measurements, or provide other compelling incentives, are part of the compliance issue and its solution. One other conclusion comes to mind regarding the evidence of what works to improve compliance: it is no mystery why compliance is so high in clinical trials. In the trials in which I have been involved, there has been a high level of communicating with, educating and valuing patients; long-term measurements of persistence are fed back to patients and sometimes special reminders are used, all of which enhance compliance.

Summary Conclusions

In this complex and perplexing area of health care, it is tempting to resort to generalities along the lines espoused by the German writer, Goethe: "Knowing is not enough; we must apply. Willing is not enough; we must do." Or to extend the mantra of patient health management, perhaps we should say: "Things can be better, and we must commit to make it happen."

However, I don't think this is enough.

Poor compliance is a real problem and needs real solutions. But this area of health care and the care gap is not easy to come to grips with. It seems uninteresting or just not worth the effort of engaging in or getting excited about. Maybe we need to develop a new way of thinking about the issue.

Along these lines, I was reminded recently by my colleague, Normand Dumoulin, of Osler's assertion that humans have an intrinisic craving for medicines. Normand, an experienced pharmacist and director of health education at Merck Frosst, sees this tendency for addiction to medicine as one end of a continuous spectrum of human behaviour. The polar opposite, or the other end of the compliance spectrum, is represented by patients who don't even get their first prescription filled. He wonders if there is something we could learn from these extremes of drug-taking behaviour that might benefit both of the extremes and result in moving the extremes toward the middle or toward more appropriate compliance behaviour.

What can we learn from this line of thought? We need to further explore ideas like this and test anything that might improve matters. In both dollar and clinical terms, fixing poor compliance would deliver an enormous windfall to the health care sector and society. Presently, it remains a complex area, incompletely understood and something of an orphan issue in accountability terms. On a positive note, however, it is important to remember that some interventions do work. We can, indeed, apply them.

They can make things better. We should be applying them and we are.

Chapter 6

ACCESS, HEALTH AND THE ECONOMY: CAN WE AFFORD ACCESS GAPS?

When I started medical school, issues such as access or economics or health costs were not in the curriculum. When I began my venture into public and population health, I was not concerned particularly with health expenditures or the economies of nations or how they were related. They just did not seem particularly important to me or my colleagues.

When I started to write this book, I did not think that this chapter would be an important one or a long one. I was wrong.

The health and the wealth of nations are intertwined and this interrelationship is important as we consider our future in the increasing globalization of our world. It is also a complex interrelationship. On average, the evidence supports a positive relationship between the health and the wealth of nations (Analysis Group/Economics 2003; Lichtenberg 1998, 2004; Nordhaus 2002). As evidence builds, I believe policy makers will increasingly act on this relationship, making policy and investment decisions that enhance their countries' competitiveness.

On an individual patient level, our access to innovative care and products may well be determined by what we can afford to pay or what insurance coverage we have. So our individual health outcomes and our potential individual contribution to the overall economy of the nation are intertwined in a microcosmic health-wealth relationship.

When health meets money, opinions are often strong and people do not always agree. There are competing, vested interests and varying opinions with regard to what and where investment should occur, what we are buying for our health dollar and who is best suited to make our financial decisions. Weighing the relationship requires us to look at both economic factors like money and market forces, and relate them to health factors like prolonged survival or improved quality of life over the long term. This presents its own problems, since few people are trained and experienced in more than one field of endeavour. Getting comfortable with the measurements and what they mean is challenging and difficult for almost everybody.

In this chapter, I will discuss some of the more recent evidence and opinions of leading thinkers to present a reasonable overview of the health-economy relationship. In particular, I will put into some perspective what we as a nation spend on health care, what we get for our money and how we might feasibly balance the costs and hoped-for benefits in the near future.

An overall perspective on the value and expenditures of health care is important for all of us as citizens if we are to understand how restricted access is contributing to care gaps. All citizens are financially covered under the provisions of Medicare for hospital and physician services, and about 85 percent of Canadians have some form of third-party insurance, either government or private payer, for out-of-hospital drug costs. When the institutional payer is balancing costs, access and quality in health care (see Figure 1.1), there is a tendency to reduce access to meet cost targets. This restriction of access to health products and services can ultimately result in less-than-optimal outcomes if a person does not receive the most efficacious therapy to reduce risk and prolong or improve the quality of his or her life.

The problem in the recent past has been that many of the decisions to restrict access to products and services have not been made in consultation with the average citizen or patient. In many cases, these decisions have not been communicated at all, and patients have been unaware of them until they have directly experienced the impact of these decisions. This relative non-transparency is troubling from the viewpoint of institutional ethics.

To act ethically, an institution must have three major characteristics. It must have a value system whose values are constant; the institution should be prepared to act on its values, not just talk about them; and it should act transparently, with all of its cards on the table. For example, to assist our partners and potential partners in understanding our value system and its application, the Patient Health team I am on at Merck Frosst has produced a statement of ethical principles that we apply to our projects and relationships. It is reproduced in Appendix A.

The following sections are intended to help the average person or patient gain a better understanding of some of the important factors that are considered when the institutions that control our health care spending make decisions. Clarifying the issues and increasing transparency in this complex and very important facet of health care will, I hope, lead to more informed and public debate regarding sustainability.

How Much Do We Spend on Health Care, and Can We Afford It?

Let's start with costs.

Perhaps the most significant economic component of health care is the cost of providing hospital, doctor or drug care. Health costs, as absolute expenditures, have steadily increased over the last few decades and are projected to continue to do so for the foreseeable future. The Canadian Institute of Health Information recently estimated health care spending for this country to be $121 billion in 2003, an increase of about 5 percent over the amount spent in 2002.

When people think about the sustainability of Canada's health system, they are often concerned by figures such as these. They wonder if health care as we have known it in the past will be affordable in the future. I believe that health care can and will continue to be affordable. I also think that care and its costs will continue to change over time in proportionate terms *vis à vis* drugs and hospitals. This belief is drawn from observations of recent changes and my belief that these relative changes reflect preferential spending on what we think are the most important, productive and efficacious elements in health care.

For example, the relative costs of physicians' services have decreased since the early 1990s, when they represented about 15 percent of total health spending in Canada. Doctors now account for less than 13 percent of total health expenditures. On the other hand, expenditures on drugs have risen as a percentage of total health costs over the same time frame, from about 12 percent in 1990 to 16 percent of the total health budget in 2003.

Hospitals remain the single most expensive line item in our health budget—about 30 percent of total costs in 2003. In the future, care is likely to increasingly shift from hospitals to community settings because of wider availability of newer, efficacious therapies, particularly new drug therapies, that can be administered in out-patient environments. These innovative therapies will improve outcomes and allow patients to avoid adverse events that used to require hospital admission in the past. With this projected shift to more community-based, out-of-hospital care, the community-based drug expenditure component of total health expenditures may increase. However, there will be an accompanying and more than off-setting decrease in related hospital-based care and costs. That is, in the immediate future, we should be able to buy better outcomes with less total cost to the health system as a whole.

When I look at health costs in relation to Canada's overall economy, I am also reassured. For example, the 2003 level of total health spending represents approximately 10 percent of Canada's gross domestic product (GDP) for 2003. To put this spending in a historical framework, in 1960 the level of spending as a proportion of the GDP was just over 5 percent. In 1970, when Medicare was introduced in most provinces, health care spending had risen to about 7 percent of GDP, reaching the 10 percent level for the first time in 1992. So relative to the GDP, the measure of the economic engine driving the country, health costs have doubled over the last forty years, but have been essentially unchanged over the last decade.

It is also helpful to realize that other countries are able to afford as much health expenditure as we do, or more. For example, in 2001, in terms of health spending indexed to the GDP, Canada's 9.7 percent spending level placed it behind the United States (13.9 percent) and Germany (10.7 percent) and just ahead of France (9.5 percent) and Japan (7.6 percent). So we are in the first rank of health spending as indexed against our economic engine, but we are not the leaders and we are not profligate.

Two differences in health spending between Canada and the United States are worth examining. These differences are increasingly recognized as important by many decision makers in each country and will very likely influence future health funding decisions in both countries.

One difference is that 40 million of the nearly 300 million people in the United States have no health insurance coverage. That is, unlike Canada, the United States does not have universal health care, but its absence is increasingly a political issue and a motivator for change. The second difference is that the proportion of health care and health research spending in Canada that comes from the private sector is relatively small compared to the United States. On the one hand, the large private-sector contribution to health care is becoming a burden for companies in the United States, which tends to make them relatively non-competitive compared to similar companies in Canada (Gross 2004).

On the other hand, the large proportion of private-sector spending on health research in the United States is giving that country an enormous advantage in attracting new investment dollars and all the other benefits of being on the leading edge of innovation, particularly in attracting the best and brightest people.

Currently, the American health sector investment totals about $45 billion a year. Canada, in contrast, is investing less than $2 billion a year in medical and health research. This is not enough to be in the front rank of the knowledge economy of the future or even the present.

Given the relatively common social values and essentially shared information environment of Canada and the United States, it seems reasonable to assume that, over time, there will be increased pressure to share a more common approach to health issues like funding and coverage. In particular, I predict that in the United States health care insurance coverage will continue to move toward universality and that funding responsibility for that care will shift more toward public sources.

In Canada, we will not willingly move away from universality of coverage. I suspect, however, there will be increasing pressures to shift costs of some care and products more to individuals or corporations in the private sector. Both private and government levels of spending on health research will have to increase in Canada if we are to reach the front ranks of health innovators in the increasingly competitive and globalized world.

In a nutshell, the health environments of Canada and the United States are likely to become more similar in the future. If this indeed occurs, the similarities may well extend beyond similar amounts of dollars (per capita) being devoted to research to similar prices being paid for services and goods obtained.

What Are We Buying with Our Health Care Dollars—Is There Value?

If we can afford, at least theoretically, what we spend on health care, the next important question is: does the money spent bring value or even a premium return?

In fact, as a nation, Canada has relatively attractive population health measures. For example, Canadians have among the lowest infant mortality rates and the highest longevity figures in the world.

Since we don't spend as much as some other countries on health, and yet have better health outcomes, some observers have suggested this is evidence that health spending and health outcomes are not related. In fact, as I mentioned in a previous chapter, during the initial cost-cutting in the restructuring of Medicare of the last decade, there was some attempt to justify the desired cost reductions by invoking this hypothesis. The evidence, at least as I understand it, is, however, very much in the other direction—health outcomes and the money we invest in striving for better ones are very much related.

The first line of evidence I became aware of was from Alberta and came during the latter part of my tenure as director of cardiology in Edmonton. Dr. Richard Plain of the University of Alberta measured the amount of public expenditures per person on health care in Alberta between 1975 and 1992. He related this measure of health costs to life expectancy of the population in the province for the same time frame. Briefly, Dr. Plain found that there was a very close and direct relation between health expenditures and length of life in Alberta. His results are outlined graphically in Figure 6.1.

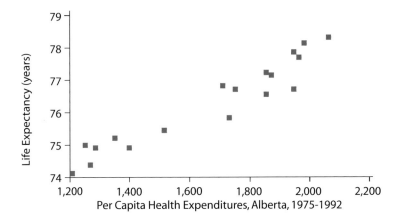

Figure 6.1: Relation of average life expectancy, in years, to average per-person health expenditures in the province of Alberta between 1975 and 1992. The per-person, or per capita, dollar expenditures have all been expressed in terms of their value in 1986 dollar amounts. Over the seventeen-year time frame, there was a direct relation between the two factors—the higher the health expenditures, the longer the life expectancy. The high degree of the interaction of dollars expended and life expectancy is reflected by the tight clustering of the individual-year data points around an invisible, nearly straight line running from bottom left to upper right in the diagram. This very high correlation, which can be expressed mathematically as $R^2 = 0.91$, suggests that expenditures and outcomes are not only mathematically related, but also causally related. Adapted, with permission, from personal communication with Richard Plain.

Subsequently, data from a variety of other countries and involving many disease states have become available and are very supportive of Dr. Plain's early findings of the societal value of investment in health care.

For example, in analysis of the introduction of new drugs and longevity in the American population between 1970 and 1991, Dr. Frank Lichtenberg of Columbia's Graduate School of Business observed a positive relationship across all diseases studied and estimated an incremental 11,200 lives saved per year for the average new drug launched during the study period (Lichtenberg 1998).

Lichtenberg has more recently expanded his studies to include analysis of similar data from more than fifty countries

(Lichtenberg 2004). In this expanded analysis, covering the period from 1986 to 2000, in both developed and underdeveloped countries, he found an incremental gain in longevity of 1.96 years among the fifty-two countries sampled, and attributed 40 percent of this gain in life expectancy to the introduction of new drugs into the countries' markets. Lichtenberg's findings indicate a direct relation between investments in innovative therapies and improvements in population health outcomes, notably increased lifespans. They are supported by similar large-scale econometric analyses of others (Cutler and McClellan 2001), including results from a recent Canadian overview (Analysis Group/Economics 2003).

Overall, the evidence suggests that spending on health services, particularly innovative services, results in improved health outcomes in the population.

This makes sense on an individual level, too. For example, it is readily accepted that, if you get pneumonia and you invest in the appropriate therapy, you are likely to avoid death and disability. Investment and outcome are linked in health care.

Linking improved health outcomes through investment to improvements in the general economy of the country at large is another challenge.

Some evolving research has, however, addressed this further step in evaluating health investments. One approach converts gains in health outcomes like longevity into dollars, a calculation referred to as the value of a statistical life. Using these standard economic values for avoided deaths or increased life expectancy, a recent overview study sponsored by a coalition of health stakeholders in the United States reported that the value of investment for every dollar spent on health care ranged from $2.40 to $3.00. That is, for every dollar spent, between $2 and $3 were returned to the economy. This represents, then, a worst-case societal return on investment ratio of 2:1 and a best-case ratio of return of 3:1. In business terms, this is very good.

Using another economic model, the value return on investment for health at the national economy level was also estimated by Nordhaus, from the University of Chicago. Taking into consideration health benefits such as prolonged lifespans for people in the population produced by innovative therapies, he suggested that the economic growth of a nation may be twice as large as the traditionally calculated growth unadjusted for the longevity benefit (Nordhaus 2002).

Is the Link between Health and the Economy Accepted in Canada?

Historically, this line of thought has not been the tradition in our country.

Increased health expenditures have traditionally been viewed as singular components and ever increasing with little visible return in economic terms related to any improved clinical outcomes. Recently, physicians, economists, politicians and others have begun to recognize the health industry as an important growth driver within the total economy of a nation, a proposition not unlike the hypothesis proposed by Nordhaus (2002).

In a speech to the Montreal Board of Trade on September 18, 2003, Paul Martin, who at the time was soon to become prime minister, suggested a blueprint for building the economy of the twenty-first century: "The key of any good strategy is to concentrate on your strengths. We need to pick segments where we can really build a competitive advantage in the global market . . . The important thing is that we move quickly to leverage our existing strengths . . . and make health care not just a powerful force in society, but a growing force in our economy."

Similar opinions have been voiced recently by academic opinion leaders and champions of health research investment in Canada. For example, Henry Friesen, chair of Genome Canada and former president of the Medical Research

Council, has stated: "It's time to see our health system not simply as a provider of health for Canadians, but as a generator of wealth for Canada. The Health and Health Care sectors should be viewed not as a cost to be borne, but as an opportunity to be explored."

The president of the Canadian Institutes of Health Research, Dr. Alan Bernstein, in a speech entitled "Advancing Health, Science, and the Economy," delivered as part of the fourth Annual Directions for Canadian Health series, said: "We need to stop viewing the health care system as a cost centre that needs to be contained and start recognizing the money we spend on health as a valuable investment in the world's largest knowledge-based sector."

All in all, research evidence and expert opinion suggest that health care and health research dollars are not just falling down some bottomless money pit with no return value to society. The evidence-based new thinking is saying that the introduction and diffusion of new therapies into any population or health care market are practical reflections of the quality ladder model of innovation. In simple terms, investment in new and innovative therapies produces advancements in outcomes over previous therapies, including greater duration and quality of life. With improvements in patients' health and life come increased economic productivity and wealth of nations. The factors of investment and outcomes, both clinical and fiscal outcomes, are directly related.

The bottom line: If you invest in health, you will benefit as a person and as a nation.

How Do Health Expenditures Relate to Access and the Care Gap?

As indicated in Figure 1.1, within the health system there is a dynamic and interrelated tension among costs, access to products and services and quality of outcomes when health care is viewed as a system.

The great management challenge in health care is finding the right or best balance of quality, access and costs for the health system and the national economy.

For example, enhancing access to a particular proven service, such as lipid-lowering drugs to patients with cardiac disease, may lead to increased cost for these drugs because of increased use. Simultaneously, however, the increased use will yield both improved quality of clinical outcomes and decreased system costs. This latter eventuality will occur because the improved clinical outcomes will include significant decreases in emergency visits and prolonged hospitalizations and their associated costs, particularly among high-risk patients.

Supply-side economic strategies, which have been dominant in the last decade in health administration in Canada, often recommend restricting access to products and services. These restrictive strategies may achieve the intended outcome of containing isolated costs of component health budgets, drug costs or physician fees, for example. This type of health administrative strategy is not, however, the best management choice when one looks from a position of system strategy designed to attain the best population health.

This is because restrictive strategies often have the unintended but adverse impact of limiting the optimum benefits of innovative products and services within the whole population. There are no qualitative interactions in biology. If something works, it tends to work for everybody. Restricting access to an efficacious therapy also restricts its benefits, or does not allow avoidance of harm, for those who don't receive it.

Within the current health care environment in Canada, where universal access is one of the principles of Medicare and a watchword in the debate, "suboptimal" or "restricted access to services" can be politically sensitive phrases and may benefit from further explanation and definition in specific areas of health care. Drugs provide a very representative case.

Historically, drugs for patients outside of hospitals were not provided for under Medicare. However, the clinical and economic value of modern efficacious drugs in our society is increasingly recognized. They have become very valuable tools to reduce chronic disease burdens. But there is little similarity from province to province, other than the general tendency to restrict or delay access, in terms of which drugs or when specific drugs are government-funded or reimbursed. It may be particularly beneficial to consider this topic in the health debate in terms of universality and equity of access to therapy as separate issues.

For example, so-called last-dollar coverage, in which the insurer becomes the provider of last resort to prevent financial disaster or non-insurability for patients with chronic and serious diseases, offers universality and equity of access in the sense that monetary thresholds could be the same for everybody. Provision would start after some defined threshold expenditure had been already absorbed by individual or other third-party resources. This does not, however, imply universality of access to all efficacious medications or other therapies.

In contrast, first-dollar insurance by a public payer or insurer could, at least theoretically, reimburse all the costs of a prescribed therapy. Optimally, to be universal and equitable, the coverage would be for all proven therapies for all important diseases and be exactly the same for all patients everywhere in the country. The interrelation of access and costs would likely make this type of coverage a cost-dominant issue. But even if such a system were operational and practical, it would not address major inequities of treatment, in particular the under-treatment of older and female patients relative to their younger and male counterparts in any given region or clinical setting. This is discussed in the following chapter.

Balancing the interrelated components of increasing demand for quantity and quality of drugs and other proven and promising therapies against their costs and against universal and equitable access to them is a complex undertaking. We have a long way to go before we can hope to arrive at a consensus in defining concepts such as equity in care. However, the practical relevance to us as citizens of these complex health and economic issues is that we must be aware of them and understand them in order to best manage them for our optimum benefit as a society and to remain competitive in the global economy. We need knowledge combined with careful evaluation of options to make the best choices for our future.

However, to answer the question posed by the title of this chapter, the consistent weight of evolving economic analyses and econometric data suggest that no country can afford restrictive access to innovative medical therapies if it aspires to be in the front rank of both health and economic outcomes in the world.

Is there any accountable and feasible health management strategy that offers, simultaneously, the best health for the most people at an affordable and best cost? Can it be put into practice? Yes, I think so. It is called patient health management.

Chapter 7

THE CARE GAP GORILLA: BIGGER GAPS FOR OLDER PATIENTS

I began my work in defining care gaps under the assumption that care was being prescribed differently for older patients compared to their younger counterparts with the same or similar medical conditions. The results from the analysis of the first cohort of 207 consecutive heart attack patients in 1987 and 1998 at the Victoria General Hospital in Halifax and the University of Alberta Hospitals in Edmonton (see Figure 7.1), and all subsequent analyses involving many hospitals in many cities, have consistently demonstrated that older patients receive less of proven therapies than younger patients.

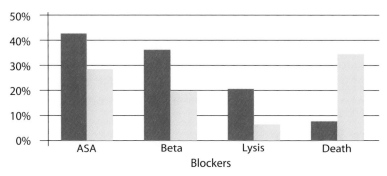

Figure 7.1 Comparison of in-hospital use of acetylsalicylic acid (ASA) or Aspirin, beta blocker and thrombolysis (clot-buster) therapies and death rates of 207 consecutive younger (less than seventy years of age, blue bars) and older (seventy years of age and older, yellow bars) patients with heart attacks, 1987–1988. Adapted, with permission, from *Canadian Journal of Cardiology* (Montague, Wong, Crowell et al. 1990).

Why practice patterns are so age-dependent remains for me a great enigma. However, it is a reality and it is meaningful for patients and their outcomes. I think its continuance is adversely prejudicing the attainment of best outcomes. With our aging population, it is likely to have an even greater negative societal impact as we go forward.

For a long time, even as I repeatedly encountered these age-discriminating patterns and outcomes, I resisted ascribing the cause of these practice patterns to any deep-seated, heuristic prescriber bias against older patients. This seemed so unreasonable a causal explanation to attribute to professionals grounded in science and principles of evidence. It may not, in fact, be the primary explanation, but I would like to suggest that you fairly consider this possibility because, after all is said and done, I keep coming back to it as a root cause.

Prescribing physicians are integral parts of our communities and our daily lives. They have value systems similar to those of mainstream society. If society is relatively undervaluing older citizens, including their quality of life and their productive potential, it seems reasonable to assume that some of this value system will be embraced and exhibited by physicians.

In other words, if society's value of older people and their contributions to important societal endpoints, such as gross domestic product and quality of life and family relationships, were to improve, the prescription of proven medical therapies to older people might also increase. To make things better, maybe we need more old people in beer commercials!

The Evidence

From a scientific point of view, older patients generally are the patient group at the highest risk from chronic diseases such as heart disease or osteoporosis. The scientific evidence also suggests that efficacious therapies have as much or more impact in the highest-risk patient groups (McAlister et al. 1999).

Presumably, this is because the cause of the illness is present to a higher degree in higher-risk patients, such as older patients. This also may mean that there is greater potential for beneficial effects from these treatments in these higher-risk patients. In other words, there is more opportunity to lower risk in a higher-risk setting.

It would seem logical, then, to set the bar lower for intervention with efficacious therapy in the higher-risk groups. Yet the repeated monitoring of prescribing patterns suggests the opposite situation is more often the case. The basic question becomes: what is this counter-intellectual pattern of practice based on? What drives it?

Although I still do not have completely satisfactory answers, I did acquire some compelling insights from the investigations led by Dr. Laurel Taylor. Dr. Taylor, as part of her PhD research, mounted a large two-part survey of physicians' intention-to-treat decisions and the underlying reasons influencing these decisions. Briefly, using a case study of heart attack standardized for all clinical variables, but for two different patient ages (fifty-four years and seventy years), Dr. Taylor and colleagues asked several thousand physicians about their patient management intentions, specifically the likelihood of performing risk-stratification tests and prescribing proven and unproven drug therapies. The results are summarized in Figure 7.2.

Physicians indicated very high intentions to use proven therapies and avoid non-proven therapies. They also intended to measure risk of future events for the patients at a high rate, particularly through the use of exercise tests and echocardiograms.

The intentions to use proven therapies were much higher than the prescription patterns usually measured by chart audits of real-world patients with the same heart attack problem. In other words, care gaps in intention are much smaller than care gaps in practice. Physicians don't quite do what they say they intend to do. Something seems to happen between the intention-to-treat decisions and the actual treatment implementation that mitigates the use of proven therapies. The big question is: what?

Interestingly, although the care gaps in intention are much smaller than the care gaps in practice, there remains an identifiable persistence of an age difference in intention to treat that is unfavourable to older patients.

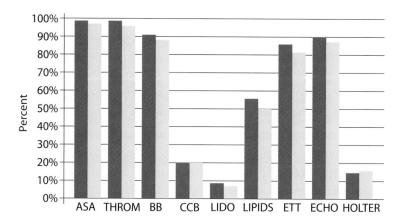

Figure 7.2: Intentions of 2,136 physicians for prescription of proven (ASA = acetyl-salicylic acid; throm = thrombolysis or clot buster; BB = beta blocker) and unproven (CCB = calcium channel blocker; LIDO = lidocaine) drug therapies and risk-stratifying tests (ETT = exercise tolerance testing; ECHO = echocardiographic measure of heart pump function; HOLTER = twenty-four-hour electrocardiographic monitoring of heart rhythm) for two representative heart attack patients, one aged fifty-four (blue bars) and one aged seventy (yellow bars). Reproduced, with permission, from PhD thesis (Taylor 2001).

These trends in intention to treat were generally consistent across all geographic areas, but varied somewhat with physicians' practice settings and specialties. For example, cardiologists and internists, as well as physicians closer to their formal training, displayed greater intentions to use proven therapies. In other words, specialists and younger physicians intend to use proven therapies more frequently than generalist physicians or older doctors.

Representative results from the second part of the Taylor survey, which analyzed factors that might influence treatment intentions for the same case study of heart attack, are summarized in Figure 7.3.

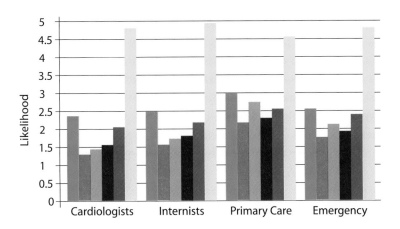

Figure 7.3: Factors influencing the likelihood that physicians will prescribe thrombolysis therapy in patients with acute heart attacks. For each specialty, physicians rated the evidence base (yellow bars) as the most important influence on treatment intention; second was age of the patient (green bars). The other influencers were: patient sex (red bars) and previous history of another heart attack (light blue bars), diabetes (navy bars) or high blood pressure (blue bars). Reproduced, with permission, from PhD thesis (Taylor 2001).

The factors influencing intention varied somewhat among the different therapies or from one drug to another. However, consideration of age as an influence was rated as the second to fourth most important factor in all management decisions for these patients with heart attack.

The dissonance arises when one realizes that the evidence base favours or at least does not discriminate against use of proven therapies in older heart attack patients (McAlister et al. 1999). Thus, if evidence is the dominant influencing factor in patient management decisions and age is consistently considered also, the intention-to-treat surveys and actual practice pattern audits should show equal or higher use of proven therapies in the higher-risk older patients versus younger lower-risk patients. But this is not the case, as the weight of prescribing data demonstrates.

To a lesser degree there are similar trends in prescription patterns based on patient sex, with females receiving less of proven therapies. However, as indicated in Taylor's analysis (see Figure 7.3), patient sex is not as likely as age to be considered as an important factor in influencing management decisions. In repeated multivariate analyses of the CQIN network, sex was never found to be an independent factor to increase risk of dying from a heart attack. Older age, on the other hand, was always associated with greater risk in a continuous manner; the older the patients, the higher the risk.

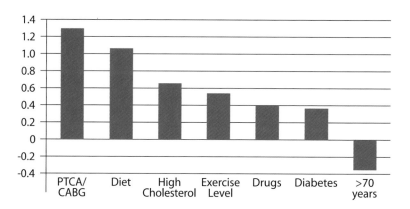

Figure 7.4: The likelihood of various clinical factors being associated with measurement of blood fat levels (for example, cholesterol) during hospital admissions for 3,304 consecutive heart disease patients. Factors rated above the zero line were positively associated with the likelihood that a patient would have his or her blood cholesterol levels measured. These included: previous patient history of angioplasty (PTCA) or bypass surgery (CABG), or previous treatment with a lipid-lowering diet (Diet), previous diagnosis of high cholesterol measurements, exercise level, or drug treatment for it (Drugs), or previous diabetes. Older age (> 70 years) was, however, linked with a decreased chance of patients having this measure of risk checked during their hospital stay. Reproduced from *American Journal of Cardiology* (The Clinical Quality Improvement Network [CQIN] Investigators 1995), with permission from Excerpta Medica Inc.

Moreover, age bias seems to extend beyond prescription of medications. It also is seen in the use of diagnostic tests to assess patient risk and prognosis. In one study of such testing patterns in heart patients, a multivariate analysis of demographic and clinical factors associated with increased likelihood of using a simple blood test to further stratify risk and refine future management of high-risk patients, older age was the only factor linked with decreased likelihood of patients receiving the test (see Figure 7.4).

Why Are Age-Related Practice Patterns Important?

Age-related practice patterns are important for two reasons. First, we may be mistaking cause for effect and vice versa. Second, the older, poorer female demographic is increasing in chronic disease populations.

In the first case, when you repeatedly measure relative underuse of proven therapies and relative over-risk for adverse outcomes in the same patient population group, you cannot help but wonder if the two variables are causally related. That is, could the consistently higher risk of older patients be caused to some degree by the lower rates of receiving efficacious therapies? And, conversely, could the higher risk of older patients be reduced substantially if their utilization levels of proven therapies increased?

I think the answers to these questions may be yes. At the University of Alberta Hospitals, where much of the early work on care gaps and closing them was defined, repeated measurement and feedback of patterns and other innovative therapeutic disease management innovations over several years was associated with closing prescription gaps.

Interestingly, however, the reduction in hospital mortality risk during the time of the improved practice patterns was essentially confined to the older patient subgroup (see Figure 7.5).

87

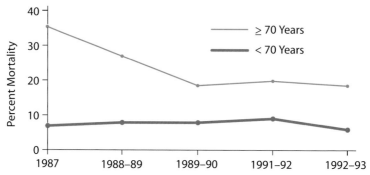

Figure 7.5: Comparison of in-hospital mortality rates of consecutive yearly cohorts of younger (< 70 years of age) and older (≥ 70 years) heart attack patients at the University of Alberta Hospitals, 1987–1993. The risk of dying among the older patients decreased from 35 percent to 19 percent between 1987 and 1990 and remained stable at this level. In contrast, the risk of dying among younger patients decreased from 7 percent to 6 percent over time. Adapted, with permission, from *Journal of Thrombosis and Thrombolysis* (Montague, Montague, Barnes et al. 1996).

This reduction occurred even though the older patients did not reach the same levels of use of the proven drug therapies as younger patients (see Figure 7.6).

The second reason for getting a better handle on the problem of age and sex treatment differences and its solution is related to the large and rapidly growing proportion of older, poorer and female patients in the chronic disease populations.

At least for heart disease, not only are there care gaps, there also appears to be a large social gap in the current demographic or distribution patterns of factors such as older age, female sex, low income and solitary living environments among heart disease patients (see Figure 7.7). In other words, the medical and societal issues regarding older patients in health care are related and important. They are the practical forest, not just a few interesting academic trees. This type of data supports the views of Pierre-Gerlier Forest that society's health policies regarding the increasing age of our population should consider related social environmental factors if we aim to optimize care, outcomes and productivity for this important segment of our society.

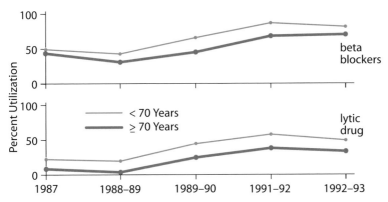

Figure 7.6: In-hospital use of beta blocker (top graph) and thrombolysis, or clot-buster (bottom graph) drugs in consecutive heart attack patient cohorts at the University of Alberta Hospitals, 1987–1993. Although the use of both proven therapies increased with time in both age groups, the older (> 70 years) patients never achieved the same level of use as the younger patients. The age-based difference, or care gap, in level of prescription of these efficacious therapies persisted. Adapted, with permission, from *Journal of Thrombosis and Thrombolysis* (Montague, Montague, Barnes et al. 1996).

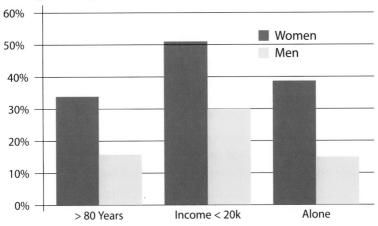

Figure 7.7: Frequency comparison of age greater than eighty years, low income and solitary living arrangements between men and women patients hospitalized with unstable angina and/or heart attacks in Nova Scotia. Female patients are older, poorer and more often alone. Adapted, with permission, from the ICONS database.

Underlying Causes

Despite being aware of the age and, to a lesser degree, the sex differences in prescribing practices and intentions for many years,

89

I remain uncertain about the underlying cause or causes. It is, however, possible to reasonably speculate on likely causes.

Perhaps there is no single cause for the apparently less-than-preferential prescription patterns in older patients. Perhaps there are valid reasons for physicians to make their treatment decisions that are evidence based, but beyond the usually considered evidence base of clinical trial results.

For example, in multivariate analyses of large populations of consecutive patients admitted to hospital for heart failure, it is not surprising to find that proven therapies such as angiotensin-converting enzyme (ACE) inhibitors are associated with increased chance of survival. After all, that is what the randomized clinical trials predicted. What is striking in these analyses is that some non-proven therapies, such as calcium channel blockers and anti-coagulants or blood thinners like coumadin, are also associated with a decreased risk of dying. This suggests that physicians, on an individual basis trying to do what is best for individual patients, are able to bring to bear experience, social context and/or other recognized or subliminal influencing evidence to make treatment decisions that are efficacious for their individual patients in their particular circumstances and time. These physicians seem to be able to draw on an evidence base that complements and adds to the available randomized trials alone.

It is possible that decisions not to treat older patients with proven therapies by the same well-intentioned doctors may also fall into this rather ill-defined evidence and experience base that goes beyond trial evidence.

Alternatively, the problem of underused proven therapies in the aged may reflect some counter-intellectual undervaluing of efficacy equity in older people. This may have been fostered by the frequent and deliberate exclusion of older patients from participation in earlier-era randomized clinical trials.

There may also be some misinterpretation or misreading of older patients' expectations to be treated equally in order to have an equal or better chance for optimal longevity and quality of life. Perhaps another way to express this latter concept is that physicians may have an unfavourable bias toward older patients that causes them to set the intervention bar too high when they are making prescribing decisions, rather than lowering the bar as the evidence would favour to obtain the best outcomes.

Many years ago, when first debating the possible causes of the age-based differences in prescription patterns, I also considered that patients themselves might contribute to the differences in care levels. I thought they might have views on the appropriateness of therapy for themselves that were non-concordant with the prescribing caregivers. Certainly, lack of physician-patient concordance on the balance of risk of disease and benefit of therapy is well described in the compliance literature as a cause of patients not persevering with prescribed therapies (see Chapter 5).

When I discussed my theories in relation to male-female care gap differences with a very competent and experienced head nurse several years ago, she said the reason for the differences was simple. Her theory, based on her experience, was that females, relative to male patients, did not complain or put their cases forcefully enough. If true, this rationale may be extended to the older patients as well since, increasingly, older patients are women (see Figure 7.7).

Dr. Ken Rockwood is professor of medicine and holder of the Weldon Chair in Geriatric Medicine at Dalhousie University in Halifax. He believes that some of these age-related differences in practice patterns may reflect physicians' confusion of chronological age with biological age, an assessment of cumulative disease burden and risk regardless of the number of years the patients have lived. He says:

As people age, they accumulate illnesses in different ways. Some lucky few have minor problems that do not much affect their lives, like cataracts, low thyroid

91

function and rashes. Other elderly people have these problems, and then a single disabling problem, like stroke or cancer. Most, however, experience a few related problems, like high blood pressure, diabetes and heart disease, and a few unrelated ones, like arthritis, constipation or progressive deafness. Some unlucky few have these illnesses, and a single disabling one.

Each of these different patterns carries with it a different prognosis, and while we would certainly view it as a care gap if best therapies were not used in the first group (those with few problems), we might even think it merciful to withhold therapy in the last group (those with many problems, some of which are disabling).

Unfortunately, when people are suddenly ill with a serious problem like a heart attack, it can be surprisingly difficult to distinguish those who are more likely to benefit from those who are less likely to benefit. Most physicians practising today have no formal training in geriatric medicine, which teaches these sorts of assessment skills—in essence how to distinguish between a person's chronological age and their biological age. As a consequence, although their intentions are good when it comes to treating older patients, the tendency is to see all old sick people as having both a high risk and a poor prognosis. This often means that many physicians withhold care because they think that it is the best thing to do.

Ironically, and unfortunately, this can mean that they withhold care from some of the patients who are the most likely to benefit.

Conclusions on the Aging Gorilla

I recognize that many of the points addressed earlier raise ethical and social issues that are difficult to resolve in one book, despite many years and lots of information to work with. Nonetheless, my strong sense is that there is an opportunity to give better care to seniors, more so than for others. They can be healthier, happier and more productive with better care on the available evidence. And the net cost is likely to be in the nation's favour if we improve the health care of our senior citizens.

Alternatively, some might argue that we may spend too much on older patients. They can easily see the tragedy of a healthy forty-four-year-old person dying suddenly of a heart attack and pre-empting the remainder of what might have been a very productive life. They feel it is somewhat less tragic if the same event occurred for a healthy eighty-four-year-old person, although it might be pre-empting an otherwise happy and productive life of many years.

In other words, it is okay to spend to foster achievement of usual life expectancies, but it is not okay to spend to exceed usual life expectancies.

To balance this type of thought process and its conclusions, I offer two observations. First, what is usual life expectancy is a shifting target. In Caesar's time, the average life expectancy was in the mid-twenties. By the early part of the twentieth century, it had increased to the mid-forties and now it is in the late seventies or early eighties. Health spending has had a large role in the increases of the past century.

Finally, age is just not a positive factor in terms of risk and prognosis in health care. On the other hand, perhaps patients should feel lucky in comparison to some other groups such as athletes, where age seems to be even more of a burden. But perhaps what I am really worried about in age-based prejudice in medical care is that the treatment decision bar may shift even further in the wrong direction.

As I write this section, Colleen Jones and her colleagues have just won another Canadian curling championship. In the morning papers there were repeated reports highlighting not only her team's unique achievement of winning this competitive event in five of the last six years, but also accounts of them being booed from the stands. They were not apparently the crowd's favourite team. When I heard or read Ms. Jones's comments on these events, she seemed to feel that the fans wanted to see someone else, someone new and perhaps someone younger, win the title. Ms. Jones is forty-four.

PART 2

THE PRACTICE—
PATIENT HEALTH MANAGEMENT (PHM)

Chapter 8

BACKGROUND AND RATIONALE
OF PATIENT HEALTH MANAGEMENT

Q. Is there any accountable and feasible health management strategy that offers, simultaneously, the best health for the most people at an affordable and best cost?
A. Yes. Patient health management is such a strategy.

Q. Can it be put into widespread practice?
A. Yes.

What Is PHM?

Patient health management (PHM) belongs to the area of health care that is most commonly called disease management. While disease management is not a new term, it has no universally accepted definition. Rather, it is often defined according to a set of characteristics. In this regard, it reminds me of the difficulty that people sometimes have in defining leadership. Many people know what it is, but they have trouble in easily defining it.

Some phrases I have often heard used and which I use to describe disease management include:

- patient-centred approach to prevention, diagnosis and therapy of illness
- drug and non-drug therapy

- collaboration and coordination of services and interventions
- shift away from isolated inputs and controls, such as bed counts or hospital closures
- monitoring, measurement and feedback of practices and outcomes
- system view of health; integration of components
- improvement of the health of whole populations
- knowledge creation and dissemination

In a comprehensive overview of the nature and relation of outcomes research and disease management written by Epstein and Sherwood in 1996, the authors outlined the types of outcome measures being developed in this evolving health arena. In particular, they indicated that the measures used in the disease management field went beyond the typical outcome measures common in clinical medicine and traditional epidemiology. These measures included things such as assessment of quality of life and economic endpoints such as quality-adjusted life years.

Epstein and Sherwood defined disease management as "an explicit systematic population-based approach to identify persons at risk, intervene with specific programs of care, and measure clinical and other outcomes" (Epstein and Sherwood 1996). These authors went on to point out the increasing importance of systematic information gathering and interpretation for determining intervention opportunities in future management of patients. They positioned this population approach to outcomes measurement and management as a key feature of modern disease management.

More recently, the Disease Management Association of America has defined disease management as a "system of coordinated health care interventions and communications for populations with conditions in which patient self-care is significant" (www.dmaa.org/definition.html).

They further characterized disease management as supporting the physician–patient relationship, emphasizing prevention, using evidence-based practices and patient empowerment, and evaluating clinical, humanistic and economic outcomes on an ongoing basis with the goal of improving health.

They also list on their Web site other representative components of disease management, endeavours such as patient self-management education to address such issues as poor compliance and routine or repeated measurement and feedback of performance data to relevant health stakeholders, including patients.

All of the concepts and characteristics outlined in these definitions are relevant and familiar. We have used all of them, particularly measurement and feedback, as major tools or interventions in our PHM projects and programs.

In my view, there is value in a broad and inclusive characterization of disease management. This approach allows for many different initiatives and players to feel welcome in and a significant part of the health care arena. It also stimulates innovation and faster adoption of best practices in the evolution of the discipline.

To boil it all down, I believe the key elements in effective disease management are an orientation toward whole communities of patients and adoption of a system view of the economic, clinical and management processes and outcomes of health care.

Perhaps above all is the belief that things can be better, paired with a commitment to act to make them better, including a willingness to measure what we do and don't do and what we receive or don't receive in return for our efforts.

At its simplest level, disease management is the focused application of resources to drive improvements in health practices and outcomes.

Why Patient Health Management?

The name Patient Health Management was applied to the group we created at Merck Frosst in late 1996 to work in the field of disease management. This particular term for our type of disease management projects was chosen for several reasons.

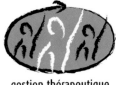

gestion thérapeutique
patient health

Figure 8.1: Logo of the Patient Health Management group at Merck Frosst.

The "patient" in Patient Health Management reminds us that patients and their interests are at the centre of health care policy and practice.

The term "health" was chosen rather than disease because it is more inclusive. It evokes continuity or a temporal spectrum in a person's life and health environment, during which one person might move from a state of wellness to disease and back again. It also highlights the prospect of being able to prevent or delay illness and disease.

Management confers the concepts of actively focusing, measuring and accounting for important factors in health care, such as therapies, their costs and outcomes. It is also meant to convey the value of non-medical skills taught in other disciplines—management schools and military staff colleges, for instance—skills such as the value of teamwork and leadership in achieving goals.

How Does PHM Relate to Traditional Medical Science and Practice?

In the PHM and the Clinical Quality Improvement Network (CQIN) projects of which I have the most experience, the principal resources were formation and maintenance of broad, community-based partnerships and implementation of facile measurement and feedback processes (see Figure 8.2).

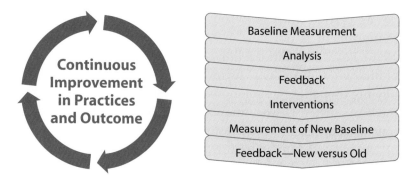

Figure 8.2: Graphic representation of the repeated measurement and feedback of practices and outcomes, the major intervention tool in PHM partnerships. This process is a feasible and powerful instrument for generating continuous quality improvement in clinical and population health. The measurements cement relationships and foster teamwork in the partnership and focus efforts toward achieving the overriding goal of making things better. The combination of a collegial, committed partnership receiving their performance data on a regular basis probably explains a large part of the so-called Hawthorne Effect, as discussed on page 107. Adapted, with permission, from *Hospital Quarterly* (Montague, Tsuyuki and Teo 1998).

The PHM projects have also utilized an assortment of data bank analyses, economic analyses, patient and professional education and reminders to elicit the desired behaviours. The projects have all focused on measuring practice patterns and health outcomes against some established benchmarks, often the results of randomized controlled trials. This benchmarking of trial evidence provides a scientific cornerstone for population health or outcomes research, a sort of moral authority or certainty that you are doing the right thing or going in the right direction.

When disease management projects are rooted in the community, as the most effective ones are, they can provide an additional sense of moral authority. They become more than academic endeavours and are deemed important enough for real people to give significantly of their time and effort toward achieving program goals and success. When this happens, it is because patients and their interests are seen as being at the centre of the endeavour.

As Epstein and Sherwood pointed out, PHM or disease management is not new or unique (Epstein and Sherwood 1996). Rather, it offers a relatively new recognition of the value of bringing to bear some areas of expertise that are traditionally not thought of as belonging to medicine in order to make medicine better. Disease management does not stand alone, unrelated to other branches of medical science.

As indicated in Figure 3.1 and in Figure 8.3, medical science and practice form a natural continuum from the basic sciences—such as physics, chemistry, molecular biology and genetics—to areas of clinical research that include randomized controlled trials or the study of pathology of disease in human subjects, and to the population health arena that embraces disciplines such as epidemiology (the study of disease in large groups of people), the economics of health care and how health outcomes are driven by clinical and policy practices.

Disease management can be considered to belong in large part to the right-hand, or outcomes, part of the health care knowledge spectrum, as represented in Figure 8.3, but it also certainly uses knowledge gained from the basic and more traditional clinical arenas, particularly the arena of randomized clinical trials.

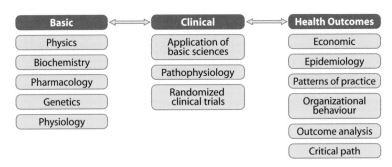

Figure 8.3: Representative spectrum of areas of expertise and investigation in medical research and practice. The more traditional areas are represented by the basic and clinical groups; the health outcomes, or population health, arena is a newer area with less traditional clusters of knowledge creation and application for medicine. Adapted, with permission, from *Canadian Journal of Cardiology* (Montague et al 1995).

The centrality of randomized clinical trials as a powerful tool for scientifically directing the medical management of patients is well established now in Canada and most of the rest of the world. The power of randomized trials is secondary to the rigorous application of statistical practices in their design and implementation. In particular, the use of randomization with large numbers of patients, along with the judicious use of exclusion criteria, has allowed investigators to minimize systematic and random bias in the definition of causative inference in the results. Consequently, the results of modern, large and simple-entry randomized trials provide a very high degree of certainty when deciding whether a new and apparently innovative therapy is truly efficacious, compared with all previously proven therapies. The large simple design also facilitates extrapolation or application of their results to a broad segment of the whole population with the target disease.

On the other hand, although randomized trials represent the benchmark or gold standard study or project design for determining truth, they are also expensive and complex. By the very nature of their robust designs, which are controlled or limited in setting, and have strict entrance criteria and specific features like formal patient education and informed consent procedures, they and their results are sometimes considered non-reflective of what would happen to patients in their daily lives outside of study protocols.

Other study designs are available for determining and relating cause and effect in clinical medicine. They range from a single observation of a phenomenon to observations of many similar phenomena, to comparisons of outcomes in patient groups before and after some intervention, with or without any control groups not receiving the intervention, through small and large single randomized trials, to groups of trials (see Figure 8.4).

The various designs can be grouped according to the degree of certainty that the study intervention truly caused the patient outcomes that were observed (see Figure 8.4). In other words, there is a hierarchy of cause-and-effect attribution among studies. In all of these study designs, truth in causal attribution can be found. However, it is important to remember that the further to the left the design falls in Figure 8.4, the higher the risk of bias affecting the result. The best approach to seeking truth in knowledge is to seek and weigh the totality of available evidence or the sum of all knowledge gained from all studies of the target disease and its modification.

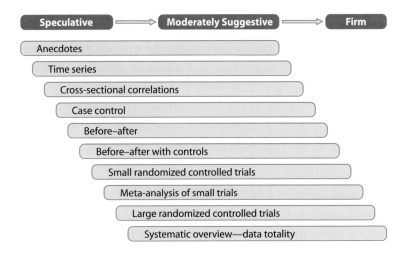

Figure 8.4: Relation of study design to the level of causal certainty that the patient outcomes observed were due to the study intervention. The study designs at the top left can discover truth in the relation of cause and effect but, relative to the study designs represented at the bottom right, have a higher chance of bias affecting the results. Studies in the middle fall in between. Adapted, with permission, from *Canadian Journal of Cardiology* (Montague et al 1995).

The Origins of Disease Management and Patient Health Management

As a medical student, I was elected to membership in Alpha Omega Alpha, the Honor Medical Society, which has the general goal of pursuing excellence in the art and science of medicine. Part of the Alpha Omega experience and a principal communication tool is its journal, *The Pharos*, which I continue to read regularly and avidly.

In the summer of 1993, an article appeared in *The Pharos* written by Kerr White, an alumnus of McGill University and member of Alpha Omega Alpha since 1949. At the time of the publication, Dr. White was retired after a very distinguished career in medicine and public health, that included stints as professor of health care organizations at Johns Hopkins University and deputy director for health sciences at the Rockefeller Foundation. Dr. White's article was entitled "Health Care Research: Old Wine in New Bottles" and dealt with the descriptive definition and historical development of the area of population health research in a most compelling way (White 1993). It remains for me a landmark paper, both knowledgeable and enjoyable and with few peers in its insight and impact. I often refer to it and re-read it. Each time, I feel proud that this influential, indeed seminal, paper on the history of outcomes research and disease management was written by a fellow Canadian.

I have used it as a roadmap here to chronicle this still evolving arena of health care.

Dr. White characterized health care research as an "eclectic field," as opposed to a traditional medical specialty. He suggested that this field of endeavour had vague boundaries within which such disciplines as epidemiology, demography, health economics, survey research, clinical decision analysis and operations research combine medical and mathematical methods to address important questions and issues such as the relation of interventions benefits to "their hazards and costs."

In Dr. White's temporal recounting, the first physician to begin to combine medicine and math at the population level was Sir William Petty in seventeenth-century England. Petty advocated measuring and comparing such things as whether doctors took as many medicines as other people in society and whether, for a given number of patients, there were differences in outcomes between patients who were cared for by physicians versus those to whom no medical art was applied.

Another early giant in the application of statistics to medical care was a French physician, Pierre-Charles-Alexandre Louis (1787–1872). Dr. Louis not only argued on behalf of the importance of measuring practices and outcomes, he also seems to have anticipated the power of randomization of intervention and control groups in assessing treatments, suggesting "the errors (which are inevitable) being the same in both groups of patients . . . mutually compensate for each other and can be discarded without sensibly affecting the exactness of the results."

Dr. Kerr White's historical review also highlights the visionary contributions of Florence Nightingale (1823–1910). Ms. Nightingale was a renaissance person, a nurse, statistician, administrator and activist in the health arena. She advocated strongly for measuring and matching care and outcomes in an attempt to get some evidence-based sense of the clinical effectiveness and cost efficiency of hospital care. Her ideas were later applied and extended by Groves in England and Codman in the United States although, as Dr. White infers, these efforts to manage by measuring practices and outcomes were not broadly or rapidly embraced and their proponents were often ostracized or marginalized.

Negative peer reaction was still apparent in the latter part of the twentieth century, although in my experience I have never seen anything approaching ostracism. Rather, initial negative reception of these ideas could be more fairly characterized as indifference based on perceived certainty that practices and outcomes are already exemplary or good enough.

One interesting story in the history of outcomes research deals with small-area variations. This phenomenon of widely variant practice patterns in apparently similar geographic areas was initially described by J.A. Glover regarding tonsillectomy rates in early twentieth-century England (Glover 1938). Since its first description, the phenomenon has been described for many other disease therapies, such as hysterectomy rates or coronary bypass rates. The causal reasons for this phenomenon are still subject to conjecture and may include intrinsic differences among physicians and/or patients and their attitudes to disease risk and its treatment benefits, not unlike those outlined above that underlie poor compliance. For some situations, however—for example, rates of angioplasty, heart surgery and other invasive cardiac procedures—small-area variation seems directly related to distance from large and sophisticated cardiac care centres.

When I first read Glover's paper, what I found most interesting was not, however, the variance of practice patterns based on geography, but the consistency of the patterns based on age—older children did not seem to receive the therapy (tonsillectomy) as frequently as younger children. That is, in the classic paper defining nearly a century ago a classic type of geography-based variation in practice patterns, there seems to be, somewhat ironically, a demonstration of consistency or homogeneity in age-based practice patterns that we have repeatedly seen in the CQIN and PHM analyses of the present and recent past.

The Hawthorne Effect

For compelling interest, nothing in the story of health care research matches, in my opinion, the phenomenon called the Hawthorne Effect. The Hawthorne Effect is ubiquitous in medical practice and disease management. It certainly can be reliably predicted to occur if the recipe of partnership and feedback of patient health management is followed. It underlies the efficacy and effectiveness of patient health management as a public health tool to make things better.

The challenge is explaining exactly what it is, despite reading the original investigators' report and many interpretive analyses of others. Here are the facts as I understand them.

Hawthorne is near Chicago. Between 1927 and 1937, researchers from what was to become the Harvard School of Business and officials from the Western Electric Company's Hawthorne plant conducted a series of experimental interventions designed to have an impact on productivity of a sample of the plant's workforce. Very interestingly, compared to how the early history of randomized clinical trials involved almost exclusively male subjects, the test subjects in Hawthorne were all women.

These women assembled telephone switches, and the series of intentional interventions focused mainly on changing the environment of the workers and comparing how fast they produced switches before and after the change. In retrospect, the interventions seem somewhat mundane. They included things such as decreasing the ambient light of the workplace and increasing it and changing the colour of paint on the walls.

To the investigators' surprise, any intervention they tried was associated with improved productivity measures, even if successive interventions were apparently opposite in direction, such as decreasing and then increasing environmental light. It appeared that the general concept of an intervention was key, as opposed to the specificity of any intervention. In clinical medicine and clinical trials, a related and similar phenomenon is often called the placebo or trial effect.

In his overview paper (White 1993), Dr. White suggested that whatever else was driving the observed improvements in the practice and productivity outcomes of making telephone switches at Hawthorne, above all, the company "cared" and "caring became an operative influence in the work environment." Although he does not elaborate on this, based on my reading of the investigators' description of the Hawthorne experiments, I think he is right.

One of the things the investigators cared about was investing the worker-subjects in a partnership. They were informed of and presumably understood the goals of the study and the processes to achieve the goals. They were also, I think, made to feel valued by being given incentives such as special uniforms, meals and health care. Above all, the subjects were made aware of the results of the measurements.

My sense is that the Hawthorne Effect is a very practical example of how human altruism can work toward making things better. Most people want things to be better. They are willing to work and contribute to improve things. This opportunity to manifest altruism in practical settings, health or otherwise, is facilitated in settings where partnerships are formed and measurements are made. Measurements provide an evidence benchmark and help to keep the partnerships together and prevent them from becoming overly concerned with process alone.

In the following chapters I chronicle some representative examples of the patient health management principles and the Hawthorne Effect in action.

Chapter 9

LEARNING EXPERIENCES: THE EPIDEMIOLOGY COORDINATING AND RESEARCH CENTRE (EPICORE), THE HEART FUNCTION CLINIC AND THE CLINICAL QUALITY IMPROVEMENT NETWORK (CQIN)

The patient health management model of health care evolved out of a number of experiences and observations. Central to them was what I saw to be the inherent value of clinical trials and using an evidence base for decision making. This chapter reviews these axiomatic experiences and traces the chain of causality through to my current patient health management initiatives. These experiences are also intended as models for others to appropriate in setting up patient health management initiatives of their own. This is how we helped make things better and how others can too.

In late September in 1987, I received a call in Halifax from Dr. Garner King in Edmonton. Dr. King was calling in his role as chair of the Department of Medicine at the University of Alberta. Now, contemporary medical university departments are usually structured into divisions such as cardiology or hematology, which specialize in specific organ systems. This model was adopted from the United States and has proven very effective in allowing Canada to be competitive with the United States over the last half century in research and training.

One of the key practical jobs of the chair of a department in a Canadian medical school is to ensure the strategic succession of the positions of divisional leaders. That is, they have to recruit people to fill planned or unexpected vacancies and to develop and support strategies for the future. Dr. King's purpose in calling me was to solicit my interest in applying for the joint position as director, leading the Division of Cardiology at the University of Alberta and the University of Alberta Hospitals.

I was interested and accepted his invitation to visit Edmonton to investigate further the possibilities of mutual interest and benefit.

I had been previously advised by a mentor and role model in such matters to take these invitations and possible opportunities very seriously. He had two reasons for this advice. One was because the people initiating the invitation were certainly taking it seriously and it was a matter of fairness that they receive equal consideration. The second reason was that a careful and systematic approach in assessing the strengths and opportunities of the possible academic marriage of an individual and an institution provided the best means to rapidly get to a feasible strategic plan if the marriage became a reality. I took this advice.

At this time, I had passed through the early and some of the middle years of a traditional academic medical career.

I was a trained clinical specialist. I had been promoted successively from assistant to associate professor of medicine at Dalhousie University and I was now to become a professor of medicine, the highest academic rank. I was being given a chance to lead and contribute to shaping the future course of a major clinical division in a major medical school. What is important for such a person in such a position to focus on to best position the group for the future?

I believed we had to focus on two things at the University of Alberta at that time to advance the academic mission and goals. The first was an educational focus. Specifically, it was to continue to concentrate on finding and training the best possible residents in cardiology. The second focus was on research. It was to build a strategy and infrastructure to attract people and financial resources in clinical research, in particular clinical trials and outcomes research.

When I went to the University of Alberta that first time to meet Dr. King and his colleagues in the university and the hospitals, I carried an outline of this two-fold strategic direction that I thought the Cardiology group should take in the future.

As events unfolded, I got the job and moved to Edmonton. The outline I presented to my potential colleagues in the Cardiology division in my initial meeting with them and later to other influential individuals in the Edmonton medical community formed the blueprint for my time in Edmonton.

Leadership

Before continuing with the chronicle of disease management experiences and institutions, I would like to relate what I learned about leadership during my early years in Alberta. It is relevant for a couple of reasons.

First, leadership is often a topic of discussion and an agenda item in teaching for those making their careers in many fields. Second, leadership is important to success in patient health management.

Certainly, it was an integral part of officer training in the army, and it is continuously reviewed and highlighted in business. When I first encountered the formal training programs in leadership as a junior officer in the army, I was skeptical. My original thought was that it was folly to think that leadership could be taught. Rather, I thought that leadership was a natural gift: either you had it or you did not. I have learned since that it is very teachable and learnable.

Leadership is an elusive concept and difficult to define, even though all of us think it is an important quality in life and feel we know what it means. A few years ago when I attended a course on leadership that included a lecture by retired American army general H. Norman Schwarzkopf, I heard a definition that has stuck with me.

General Schwarzkopf suggested that the essence of leadership was "getting others to do something they would otherwise not do." He went on to name other characteristics of a good leader, including the importance of having a durable value system and being faithful to it. This in turn, reminded me of another statement, made by Mother Teresa, who for many years led efforts to look after the poor, diseased and dispossessed of Calcutta. She said: "We are not called to be successful; we are called to be faithful."

At another leadership course I attended, I was asked to visualize the best leader I had ever met and to list his or her principal characteristics. This was an easy task for me because of my exposure to Dr. Garner King. He was the best and most successful leader I have encountered in my various careers. At the heart of his value system were the goals and aspirations of the University of Alberta, particularly the pursuit of excellence in academic medicine. He was very faithful to this goal, to the point of personal sacrifice of time and effort to contribute to others' shared pursuit of the goal. He looked after his troops.

In his case he was successful in no small part because he was so faithful to his value system and it showed. His obvious commitment to others, particularly the great joy he took in their accomplishments, encouraged people to do what they otherwise might not have done.

Three of Dr. King's principal hypotheses for effective leadership were to pick the best person for any particular job, communicate the vision and then provide all possible support, as well as continued communication, to assist that person to attain the vision and mission.

I have tried over the years to emulate some of the leadership skills and guidelines I observed in Dr. King. Principally and practically, this was by trying to find the best possible people to lead the implementation of the blueprint for our future in cardiology. In terms of evolving the cardiology residency training program at the University of Alberta, I got lucky twice.

Dr. Norman Davies became the first leader of this important divisional activity during my tenure. He was succeeded in mid-1991 by Dr. Dylan Taylor. Both of these individuals combined the best the profession has to offer. They were exemplary in patient care and had a vision of the importance of training those who would come after us. Moreover, they were sensitive to the needs and aspirations of young physicians in training and had incredible skill in two-way communication with their students. They were leaders in Dr. King's mould. They were faithful and they were successful.

As I moved into the field of population health, particularly the partnership-measurement model of patient health management, I was reinforced in my beliefs in the essential value of leadership skills to succeed. It is truly a leadership challenge to form a community-based partnership and keep it focused on the primary goal of closing a care gap over the long term.

Leadership is important in interventional epidemiology, and it cannot be taken for granted, but it can be taught and learned.

Institutions

Three very important institutions in my professional life arose from the initial blueprint for developing outcomes research and disease management capabilities at the Division of Cardiology at the University of Alberta.

Chronologically, these institutions developed in the following order: the Epidemiology Coordinating and Research Centre, the Heart Function Clinic and the Clinical Quality Improvement Network (CQIN). In retrospect, I can appreciate the logic of the sequence. However, the thoughts and drivers that led to their development were, I think, occurring simultaneously to me at that time. To some degree I still think of them as very much related in time and rationale.

The Epidemiology Coordinating and Research (EPICORE) Centre

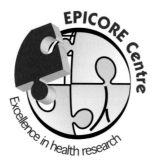

Figure 9.1: The logo of the Epidemiology Coordinating and Research Centre of the Divison of Cardiology of the University of Alberta.

By the mid-eighties, before moving to Edmonton and the University of Alberta, I had begun to get experience in large randomized clinical trials while still at Dalhousie University. I was fortunate in entering this area of medicine at an equally fortunate time. Many promising heart disease therapies were becoming available for testing—products of the basic science drug-development pipelines. And several groups were keen on developing and popularizing randomized controlled trials to test their efficacy.

The Trials Division of the Heart, Lung and Blood Institute of the National Institutes of Health (NIH), based in Bethesda, Maryland, was at the forefront of the testing for cardiac drugs. In no small measure, the emerging pre-eminence of this group was due to the presence of Dr. Salim Yusuf. He had been recruited to the NIH following extensive training in cardiology, epidemiology and trials design acquired while obtaining his D.Phil. at Oxford University in England. At Oxford, Dr. Yusuf had been significantly influenced by the ideas of the leading mathematician and bio-statistician, Richard Peto.

Peto had developed many of the modern concepts underlying the power of the large, simple trial design while working in cancer research.

My first exposure to this kind of medical research was as one of the investigators in an NIH-sponsored trial called SOLVD. SOLVD is the acronym for the Studies of Left Ventricular Dysfunction. It was a trial of medical therapy in patients who had damage to their heart muscle, most often from heart attacks; some of the patients had symptoms and some did not. SOLVD was designed as a large, simple trial with over 7,000 patients enrolled. SOLVD was a positive trial in that the drug therapy tested was found to significantly prolong life and reduce hospitalizations and other important clinical risks (the SOLVD Investigators 1990, 1991, 1992).

There were originally twenty-three medical centres enrolling patients and composing the majority of the steering committee overseeing the design, implementation and communication of SOLVD and its results. Twenty of these clinical centres were located in the United States; one was in Belgium and two were in Canada (the Montreal Cardiology Institute and Dalhousie University's Division of Cardiology in Halifax). The other major institu-tional players on the steering committee were the project officers from the NIH, led by Dr. Yusuf, and the data-coordinating centre, the Department of Biostatistics of the University of North Carolina, led by Dr. Edward Davis.

I learned much from my SOLVD experiences. However, the key value I obtained from SOLVD lay in observations of its infrastructure, process and governance. I understood how they were vital to the success of such large, multiple-partner, population-oriented initiatives designed to answer simple but important health questions. What impressed me most was the critical value of the coordinating centre, not only to the successful acquisition, quality assurance, analysis and propagation of the study's data, but also as a recognizable centre of excellence and visible magnet to attract other new projects.

As I was Alberta-bound to apply for the leadership position there, these observations led me to develop a practical keystone proposal. This was to develop a study and data-coordinating centre that would support the capacity of the Division of Cardiology to develop and coordinate its own trials and outcomes research and to serve as such a centre for others.

This idea was ultimately accomplished by attracting Dr. Pentti Rautahrju and some key members of his research team from Dalhousie University to the University of Alberta. Dr. Rautahrju became the initial holder of the Heart and Stroke Foundation of Alberta chair in cardiovascular research, and he and his team became the initial core leadership and investigators of the Epidemiology Coordinating and Research Centre (EPICORE).

Simultaneously, Dr. Koon Teo, formerly chief resident in cardiology at the University of Alberta, took up postdoctoral training in epidemiology and clinical trials under the tutelage of Dr. Yusuf at the NIH. Dr. Teo subsequently returned to Edmonton and our division and, following the departure of Dr. Rautahrju to a new position at Bowman Grey School of Medicine at Wake Forest University, succeeded to the position as director of EPICORE.

Another key recruit in the early days of EPICORE was Dr. Diane Catellier, a graduate in mathematics with a strong interest in biostatistics. She went on to do her master's and doctoral degrees in biostatistics at the University of North Carolina under the supervision of Dr. Edward Davis. Dr. Catellier's increasing knowledge and unfailing good judgment were key factors in setting a standard of excellence for the initial and all subsequent studies managed by EPICORE.

In the early years of EPICORE, we helped design and participated in several important clinical trials of heart disease therapy, including SOLVD, the Digitalis Investigation Group (DIG) trial of digoxin for patients with heart failure (The Digitalis Investigation Group 1996, 1997) and the Heart

Outcomes Prevention Evaluation (HOPE) study of patients at high risk from heart disease (The HOPE Study Investigators 1996, 2000).

EPICORE also became one of the founding members of the Canadian Cardiovascular Collaboration, a network of like-minded individuals and research centres in Canada, who realized the value of partnership and teamwork in effectively competing in the modern world of clinical trial design and implementation (The Canadian Cardiovascular Collaboration 1995).

Of perhaps greatest importance, however, regarding one of the initially proposed goals when forming EPICORE was the genesis of SCAT, the Simvastatin/Enalpril Coronary Atherosclerosis Trial. This innovative Canadian multi-centre randomized clinical trial of two promising drug interventions for high-risk heart patients was conceived, designed and co-ordinated through EPICORE. One of the major innovations in this unique trial was the simultaneous testing of two separate drugs in one study (Teo, Burton, Buller et al. 1997; Teo, Burton, DeAmeida et al. 1997; Teo, Burton, Buller et al. 2000).

Dr. Teo remembers that time:

When I returned to the University of Alberta in June 1990, after spending two years at the National Heart Lung and Blood Institute in Bethesda, Maryland, I felt ready to take on the exciting challenges in helping to set up the clinical trials coordinating activities at the EPICORE Centre.

There were several incentives for setting up the clinical trials operations quickly. One was the SCAT trial. Another was functioning as a regional coordi-nating centre for the joint National Institutes of Health–Veterans Affairs DIG Trial. In addition, the Division of Cardiology was keen to start other local initiatives, one of the first being a randomized trial of the value and safety of re-using cardiac catheters. Subsequently, we went on to act as the regional co-ordination centre for a very large and important international trial in heart disease, the HOPE trial.

The most important project at that time was, however, SCAT. Prior to my return, Dr. Norman Davies had prepared the ground. This included attracting an industry sponsor and preparing an application to the Medical Research Council of Canada for companion or matching sponsorship. The main outcome measure in SCAT was to examine the effects of drug therapy on the walls of the heart arteries. This made it necessary to be able to measure the inside of the arteries in a reliable way. Under the guidance of Dr. Davies and subsequently Dr. Jeffrey Burton, we achieved this capability in what is termed quantitative angiography and we had the additional intention of using this technology as a support facility for other trials. At the same time, we were beginning other outcomes research studies, which subsequently led to the development of the Clinical Quality Improvement Network.

It all began with the concept of a health outcomes research coordinating centre. Without the technical and personnel resources of EPICORE, it is unlikely any of these important initiatives would have been realized.

In addition, EPICORE served as the data-coordinating centre for the investigations that began in the Heart Function Clinic and, as mentioned by Dr. Teo, also provided support to the Clinical Quality Improvement Network (CQIN), the network of clinical investigators that was formed to study and improve the population effectiveness of proven therapies for major heart diseases.

EPICORE continues today under the leadership of Dr. Ross Tsuyuki, a charter member of CQIN and the Canadian

Cardiovascular Collaboration. Dr. Tsuyuki offers the following assessment of the recent past and likely future roles of EPICORE:

The EPICORE Centre has continued in its evolution. When I took over from Dr. Teo in 1999, I asked the staff "What do you think we do, and what do you think we should do?" Overwhelmingly, the response was that we provide high-quality methodology and research support for health care investigators and we should continue to do so.

We defined our mission statement: To serve the faculty and our community by generating new knowledge in the areas of health and health care through the design, execution and analysis of clinical trials, health outcomes research and epidemiologic studies (www.epicore.ualberta.ca). We have continued in this role and have extended our research support to dozens of investigators from several universities and communities, particularly community-based pharmacists.

This evolved as follows. In 1996, we were pondering the results of a study that showed low rates of assessment and treatment of risk factors, particularly blood levels of cholesterol, in patients at high risk for heart disease (The Clinical Quality Improvement Investigators 1995). In order to improve treatment of these patients, we realized the need to bring the state of this situation to the community. Around that time, the Canadian Pharmacists Association was highlighting the fact that patients see their community pharmacist five to eight times more frequently than their family physician. Going through a pharmacist thus seemed like an excellent opportunity to reach patients at high risk for heart disease.

This resulted in the creation of the Study of Cardiovascular Risk Intervention by Pharmacists

(SCRIP). SCRIP was a randomized clinical trial of dedicated community pharmacist intervention, compared to usual care, on cholesterol risk management (Tsuyuki et al. 2002). Fifty-four community pharmacies in Alberta and Saskatchewan participated in the study, where patients at high risk for heart disease were identified and approached by their pharmacist. If they were in the test group they received a full assessment by their pharmacist, including a measurement of their blood levels of cholesterol. These patients were then referred to their family physician with explicit advice on [the] next steps, based on the updated assessment of their risk level. The results of the intervention improved care in more than 50 percent of the patients.

In a similar follow-up trial, called SCRIP-plus, pharmacists provided education on cholesterol and cardiovascular disease, and facilitated communication with the patient's family physician (Tsuyuki et al. 2004). After six months of follow-up, patients' cholesterol levels dropped by about 13 percent, and about one third of the patients reached their cholesterol target levels.

This very positive impact encouraged us to further pursue the role of the community pharmacist in helping patients receive optimal therapy and ultimately led to the formation of the Centre for Community Pharmacy Research and Interdisciplinary Strategies (COMPRIS), within the framework of the EPICORE Centre, in order to facilitate the focus on community-based health research.

The Heart Function Clinic

Figure 9.2: Logo of the Heart Function Clinic of the University of Alberta Hospitals.

Of all the initiatives I have been involved in throughout my medical career, my association with the Heart Function Clinic of the University of Alberta Hospitals has given me the most satisfaction and professional gratification.

This clinic was established late in September 1989. It came into being for a couple of practical reasons.

First was the growing need to manage the continuously increasing number of patients with congestive heart failure. Congestive heart failure, often referred to as CHF, is the failure of the heart in its pump function to effectively receive used blood as it returns from the other body organs, get it oxygenated in the lungs and push it out once again in a constant cycle, repeating at approximately seventy times a minute, every minute of life. Heart failure is most often the result of one or more injuries, such as heart attacks, to the muscle of the heart's pumping chambers, the ventricles.

The principal consequences that patients notice because of deterioration in their heart's pumping ability are shortness of breath and fatigue.

Heart failure is a growth industry in cardiology, in part because of the aging population and because all adult heart diseases are age-related. It is also growing because many of the new therapies in cardiac medicine over the last two decades have been very efficacious in limiting the damage from any single acute heart attack, but they may contribute to a situation in which a patient continues to survive with a somewhat injured pump. As this cycle is repeated, the degree of damaged muscle in the heart accumulates and the symptoms and outlook worsen.

Simultaneously with the increased number of heart failure patients over the last two decades came ever-increasing limitation of hospital resources, particularly limited availability of in-patient beds and nurses to meet the increased demand. Thus, it became imperative to find some new, innovative and effective way to diagnose, treat and monitor these often ill and incapacitated patients with heart failure. The old way of treating heart disease with frequent and prolonged hospitalizations was no longer tenable.

There were some other, more positive, reasons as well. We recognized that a concentrated clinic to register and treat patients with heart failure would provide a ready source for possible patient recruitment into clinical trials like SOLVD. This was more than just an academic consideration. By 1989, when the Heart Function Clinic began to enrol patients, we had also begun to realize the power of the Hawthorne (or trial) Effect. Patients in clinical trials, by and large, find the experience very positive and rewarding. They like participating in trials and tend to do better than other patients and better than they would have if they hadn't joined the trial.

Another opportunity provided by our trials experience in managing heart failure was the availability of highly trained and experienced nurse clinicians. These nurses became the backbone of the clinic. In particular, they provided an invaluable link between the traditional hospital-based team of doctors, nurses, pharmacists and dietitians and the emergence of a family-based care team that was fostered by the new emphasis on out-patient management of the patients. And space was available in the hospitals for development of outpatient services, so we began with the principal goals of bringing intensive, comprehensive, evidence-based care to patients with heart failure in an out-patient setting and, consequently, improving their outcomes.

We used available hospital resources, including space as mentioned, but also relevant booking, investigation and consulting resources. We also used facile tools such as pocket guidelines that outlined the at-the-time, evidence-based template for comprehensive management of patients with heart failure (Appendix B).

We were successful in attaining our goals, as indicated by the measurements on comparative survival and patients' perceptions of quality of life from the early days of the clinic's existence (Figures 9.3 and 9.4 in Montague, Barnes, Taylor et al. 1996; and Figure 9.3 in Montague, Sidel, Erhardt et al. 1997) and confirmed in similar analyses later in the clinic's experience (McAlister et al. 1999).

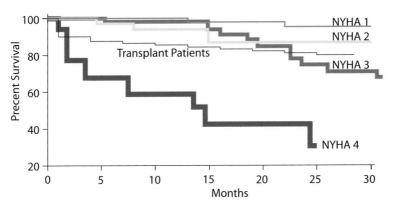

Figure 9.3: Survival patterns of 111 patients managed in the Heart Function Clinic of the University of Alberta Hospitals between 1991 and 1993, compared to the average survival for Canadian heart failure patients treated with heart transplants in the same era. NYHA refers to the New York Heart Association functional classification of patient symptoms. NHYA functional class 1 means patients had no significant symptoms or limitation in their physical capabilities at the time of entry to the clinic, despite significant damage to their heart muscle; class 2 indicates patients who had mild limitations of physical ability; class 3, moderate limitation; and class 4, severe limitation. Many of the patients in NYHA class 4 had symptoms of fatigue or shortness of breath at rest. In this analysis, survival of the heart failure patients in the clinic was very much related to limitation of physical ability or symptomatic state— the greater the limitation, the lower the survival rate. Over the short term—that is, for at least two years—patients with mild and moderate disability treated medically fared better than patients who received transplants. Adapted, with permission, from the *Canadian Journal of Cardiology* (Montague, Barnes, Taylor et al. 1996).

Knowledge Creation

The Heart Function Clinic experience and opportunity certainly increased knowledge of heart failure, its treatment, natural history and evolution. Such clinics are now common across North America and, based on a recent report in the literature (Butler et al. 2004), the prognosis of patients with heart failure managed in these clinics continues to improve. This continuous improvement in survival is, in no small way, due to the focus these clinics have placed on rapidly adopting and continuously improving utilization of proven therapies in this patient population. For example, over the first three years of operation, the use of angiotensin-converting enzyme inhibitors and beta blockers in the clinic at the University of Alberta Hospitals was 87 and 23 percent, respectively (Montague, Teo, Taylor et al. 1998). In comparison, the recent report from the Vanderbilt Heart Failure Program showed that the use of these same two efficacious medications had risen to 93 and 73 percent, respectively (Butler et al. 2004).

These life expectancies for patients with heart failure were not the norm in 1989. As it became evident that comprehensive, intensive and evidence-based care was practical and likely efficacious in prolonging life for patients with heart failure (see Figure 9.3), a new idea—what I came to call "appropriateness of care"—began to occur to us.

As Kerr White points out in his historical review of the genesis of outcomes research and disease management, appropriateness is frequently mentioned as an outcome measure of interest (White 1993). The problem from a practical viewpoint for many people is in defining or characterizing the terms of reference for determining what is appropriate. What is one person's sense of appropriate treatment is not necessarily the same for everyone. It is one of those areas in health care, such as the relative importance of the various causes of the care gap (Figures 3.3 and 3.4), in which opinions seem very much related to which seat one is occupying at the health care debating table.

I began to wonder and search for some evidence-based way to define appropriateness of medical treatment, using heart failure as the disease model (Montague, Barnes, Taylor et al. 1996).

In the early 1990s my concept of appropriateness in treatment was essentially equated with efficacy of treatment. "Efficacy," in turn, meant "proven" in a large randomized clinical trial.

In acute heart disease care—that is, for patients who have heart attacks and acute unstable angina—the most inappropriate care pattern was, and probably still is, undertreatment with many of the proven therapies, particularly among older patients (see Figure 7.1).

In heart failure care, on the other hand, we were prescribing heart transplantation as an efficacious therapy without proof from randomized trials, a sort of overprescription of non-proven therapy. The presumption of efficacy for heart transplantation in treating severely ill heart failure patients, without trials' evidence of proven efficacy, was, however, understandable. In the 1980s and early 1990s, survival with severe heart pump damage was poor and was obviously improved for patients receiving a new heart in transplant programs. Physical function and quality of life markedly improved with transplantation for these severely ill patients. The differences in prognosis and life quality between medical care only and medical care plus transplantation were so great that a clinical trial was not needed to prove there was a difference.

When, however, we began to measure the survival data from our medically-treated Heart Function Clinic patients (see Figure 9.3) and found that survival for many medically-treated patients was competitive with the survival data of patients receiving transplants, it forced us to reconsider and redefine what was "appropriate" therapy for these patients. As I read the more recent and improved survival statistics from the analysis of similar patients by Butler and colleagues (Butler et

127

al. 2004), I recognized a similar consideration being forced upon them.

While it is certainly reasonable to make efficacy one of the principal criteria in defining appropriate treatment, the experience in the heart failure world over the last decade suggests that the relative efficacy of various treatments in a particular disease should be continuously reviewed. And beyond efficacy, other factors such as cost and access should be considered when assessing the appropriateness of therapy. For example, even if heart transplantation remained markedly greater in efficacy than all usual and proven medical therapy for patients with heart failure, it would never have become an effective (or appropriate, perhaps) therapy from the population viewpoint. Each transplant and its management are very costly. And with heart failure having an occurrence rate of 1 percent of the whole population, access or availability of a donor heart becomes an issue; potentially 1 percent of the population would have to die to become donors for the heart failure group. The net societal benefits would be zero in people terms and negative in dollar terms.

From this population viewpoint, acetylsalicylic acid, or Aspirin™, might be considered the benchmark of appropriate therapy, at least for high-risk patients with underlying atherosclerosis in their arteries and a history of acute heart or stroke symptoms. It is efficacious in preventing recurrence of symptoms; it is affordable and almost everybody can take it.

My colleagues and I continue to struggle with how to best define appropriate therapy for specific conditions, most recently bringing evidence of risk status of patients into the calculations (see Figure 4.4). We will continue to evolve our thinking as we continue to accrue experiences. However, I am not sure I would have entered this important arena at all without the experience and knowledge gained in the Heart Function Clinic.

Another example of knowledge gained from clinic experience was related to the accumulation of numerous patients who, prior to their attendance at the clinic, were often admitted to hospital with worsening symptoms of their heart disease for prolonged periods. After attending the clinic, these patients began to experience long periods of life outside of hospital with improved quality of life. After about four years, there were patients who, after long periods of symptom reduction or remission, began to redevelop symptoms. At first consideration, we thought these symptoms, such as chronic cough, were a return of clinical signs and symptoms of their heart failure or possibly side effects of their medication. In due course, however, things became clear and defined.

Historically, heart failure patients tend, overwhelmingly, to die from worsening of their heart disease. We noticed that with remission or reduction in heart failure symptoms and signs, and improving survival, some patients' symptoms of fatigue and/or shortness of breath were, in fact, due neither to their heart disease nor their medications; they were due to another non-heart disease. In particular, we noticed that cancer was often developing. This anecdotal experience from a small number of patients stimulated us to mount a larger study with partners in the Clinical Quality Improvement Network of the specific causes of death among heart failure patients (Ackman et al. 1996).

As suggested by the anecdotal evidence, we found that, although heart disease continued to be responsible for most deaths among this patient population, non-heart-related causes were responsible in about a third of the deaths. Cancer was the leading cause of non-cardiac death, followed by pneumonia and lung diseases. This information confirmed our earlier suspicions from a few observations and, moreover, it gave us greater certainty in modifying or reinforcing everyday practices in the clinic. For example, we became more vigilant in managing infections and striving to protect lung function through practical interventions such as regular flu vaccinations.

The congregation of patients with heart failure led to other insights. One very interesting one came from a study that assessed which non-heart medications heart failure patients were taking and compared the findings to age, sex and socially matched control subjects without heart failure (Ackman et al. 1999). Briefly, we found that more than half of heart failure patients, whose average age was in the mid-sixties, were taking one or more non-prescription drugs, most frequently anti-inflammatory or pain-relief medications. However, so were the control subjects who had no heart failure. The only significant differences we found were a higher use of nutritional supplements and a lower use of drugs that might have negative side effects in the heart patients. Both of these differences were felt to be in line with education they received from the clinic. These patients, in fact, were taking better care of themselves, and the use of nutritional supplements and the non-use of drugs that might have negative side effects were proof of it. These patients were practising "appropriate self-prescription," to use a controversial term.

We felt it was important to disseminate this knowledge through the usual academic avenues of publications and presentations. We also shared some of our principles and practices, such as clinic infrastructure and processes and patient education materials, with other like-minded organizations. As well, we created an outreach program to bring physicians and nurses from other communities to the University of Alberta Hospitals so they could see first-hand how the clinic was operating.

This was a natural initiative to take on since none of the features of the clinic's operation were complicated or required extensive training beyond general medical training and experience. In my judgment, we were only partly successful in this educational initiative. It did, I believe, help some people and centres to start up their own clinics. But some visitors became discouraged when they visited us. Often these people were from smaller communities that were experiencing withdrawal or downsizing of many of their medical, nursing, dietitian and pharmacy resources during the early 1990s. They thought that it was a great idea for the university hospitals, but impractical for them because they had no help devoted to out-patient-focused care at that time. Nonetheless, we pressed on.

Hope with a Small "h"

I believe Dr. White's caring concept can be extended to another human value—hope. In the context of medical and health partnerships such as patient health management initiatives, they are, I believe, related and form at least part of the Hawthorne Effect as it exists in medicine.

The best example I can offer of this relationship is what I observed during my time as a physician in the Heart Function Clinic and Heart-Lung Transplant Clinics of the University of Alberta Hospitals. During the late 1980s and early 1990s, my colleagues and I were striving to improve the quality and duration of life for patients with congestive heart failure, which was and remains an important and serious burden of illness for Canadian society.

Patients with heart failure are often very ill, with many symptoms that limit their ability to function at a level they associate with happiness or fulfilment. The primary thrust of the Heart Function Clinic patient management processes was to improve life duration and quality for these patients by increasing the use of evidence-based medical therapy in a communication-rich out-patient setting. Caring was very visible in this setting, I believe, in no small measure through the medical skills and bedside manner of a small core of outstanding nurses. The formula worked; hospitalizations decreased and functional status of patients increased.

At the suggestion of the hospitals' quality-improvement team, we tried to get a handle on patients' perceptions of their quality of life by using some simple methods. We used a ladder of life model as one measurement tool. In this device, the best possible quality of life is scored at 10; the worst possible is at 0. Patients were asked to rate their life quality on this 0-to-10 scale as current clients of the Heart Function Clinic, then to rate the level in the year before they joined the clinic and, lastly, to forecast what it might be in the upcoming year. Repeated applications of this survey to various cohorts of attending patients produced similar results (see Figure 9.4).

Not surprisingly, the patients' perceptions of their quality of life improved with their participation in the clinic. More unexpected, however, was the expectation of a continuing improvement to achieve even greater quality of life in the future, such as in the next year. When I thought about this situation, two things struck me as important. First, these very ill

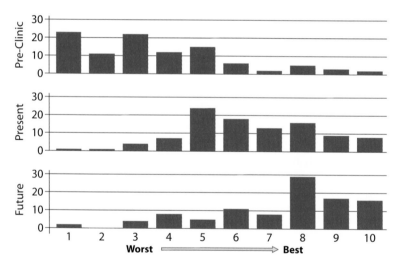

Figure 9.4: Percent distribution of quality of life perceptions among patients in the Heart Function Clinic of the University of Alberta Hospitals. On average, the patients felt things were better than they used to be and sensed, moreover, that they would likely be even better in the future. This latter sense of a better future may well reflect patients' optimism or hope, even though they have a serious disease and a prognosis that is traditionally associated with a high risk of dying in the near future. Adapted, with permission, from *American Journal of Managed Care* (Montague, Sidel, Erhardt et al. 1997).

and mostly older patients did not seem to be aware of or believe in the terrible prognosis usually associated with their heart failure diagnosis. Second, the reason for their optimistic outlook was that they had hope.

We extended these analyses to patients with heart failure who were being managed in the Heart and Lung Transplant Clinic of the University of Alberta Hospitals as well and found very similar results—attendance at these clinics, with their focus on evidence-based, out-patient-delivered care by a team that involved the patients and their families in close communication, was associated with improved outcomes and particularly a sense of improved quality of life.

As we were observing the improved clinical outcomes compared to historic norms, I began to consider that the Hawthorne Effect was instrumental in generating some of the improvements, including increased survival and better perceptions of life quality. Specifically, I thought it came from some interrelated combination of caring by the clinic staff and the patients' hope.

Einstein once commented on how he evolved his theories of relativity. Because he was the sole author, many people thought that his ideas were uniquely his own and that he was the sole source of his incredibly complex, robust and farsighted theories of how our universe works. But Einstein disabused them of this notion. Rather, he pointed out, he had benefited from those who went before him, people such as Newton and Lorentz. "They served as material for my thoughts," Einstein said (Clark 1971).

The more I trace these paths to knowledge and inquiry in patient health, the more I realize how our innovations and advances are incremental, too. Like Einstein, we are, to some degree, rediscovering the past and standing on the shoulders of giants to see new horizons.

The patients' hope that we were intuiting from our Heart Function Clinic experiences of the last decade (see Figure 9.4) and invoking as a contributor to improved outcomes is very similar to the phenomenon that was referred to by Osler a century ago as the "faith that heals" (Osler 1910) and more recently by Dr. Jerome Groopman (Smith 2004). Both of these physician-writers relate patients' spiritual state to the outcomes of their illnesses.

As elucidated by Dr. Groopman, "True hope is clear-eyed. It sees all the difficulties that exist and all the potential for failure, but through that carves a realistic path to a better future." It is not "a magic wand" (Smith 2004). This realistic description of patient hope is very similar to what I had observed from my experience in the Heart Function Clinic. Hope in this sense is no substitute for a more traditional, efficacious and proven medical therapy. It is more of a complement to traditional therapy that can contribute to improved outcomes. It is real and it is valuable.

In order to further explore our clinic's operation to help explain and perhaps even improve the perceived better quality of life associated with patient attendance at the Heart Function Clinic and, in particular, their faith and hope for an even better future despite their high-risk status, our colleagues in the Total Quality Management group at the hospitals designed and carried out several detailed patient quality-assessment analyses. This was a difficult endeavour, as it turned out. I have likened it to attempting to quantify a non-quantitative, or qualitative, value.

Many variables were assessed, including the location of the Heart Function Clinic in the hospital, its distance from the patient parking lot, the bedside manner of nurses and patients and what the patients appreciated most and least in their clinic experience and encounters. In repeated analyses, the most important thing to the patients in terms of providing them with satisfaction was the information about their disease, its treatment and outlook that the clinic staff gave them and their families. Patients valued the information they received from physicians most of all.

This latter finding was somewhat unexpected, for me at least. I knew we had some of the best nurses in the country working in the clinic. They were very experienced, knowledgeable and caring. I expected them to be rated as the highest value asset in the clinic. However, I interpreted the patients' view as indicative that physicians' knowledge was of a higher order than that of anyone else. Combined with the evolving concepts of the value of hope to patients, these additional insights generated three practical changes in our patient management process.

As a consequence of recognizing the great value of education in contributing to patients' quality of life, we began to systematically review our patient education tools and initiatives. We developed user-friendly booklets explaining the principal malfunction of the heart when it failed to pump normally. This included explanations that related directly to patient symptoms and signs of a failing heart, such as fatigue, shortness of breath, swollen legs and weight gain. A companion booklet focused on the treatment of heart failure, particularly the hoped-for benefits, as well as the side effects of medications. Through these efforts, we greatly expanded patient involvement in their care. This commitment to patient education was later applied to newsletters and e-communication tools as a means to support and cement the partnerships of large disease management projects like ICONS.

The second improvement stimulated by the patient satisfaction surveys was a commitment to reinforce a positive physician bedside manner in the clinic's interaction with patients. Since patients rated the information exchange so highly, I thought it very important to match the value they put on it by visibly recognizing their interest. This was managed by doing very simple things such as smiling when entering the patients' rooms and actively displaying a sense of caring by seeking patient input and opinion on things like changes in symptoms and treatment.

The third commitment related to the patient hope issue. When we were beginning to recognize how important hope or a positive vision of the future was to patients' perceptions of their quality and duration of life, the average age of our Heart Function Clinic patients was about seventy years. These patients had hope for the future even though they were aware of their on-average poor prognosis. These perceptions of themselves and their future did not square with the fact that older patients often may not get the same practical consideration as younger patients to receive rapid proven therapy, perhaps in part just because they are older. I resolved to try never to marginalize patients because of their age. If older patients care about and hope for the best future, so should their doctors. There should not be a gap in care decisions based on age.

Again, this reinforcement of the human side of the care covenant was not new. It was very similar in its goal to the attitude embodied by the staff of Johns Hopkins Hospital who have worn buttons displaying the message: "Caring is part of the cure" (White 1993).

Overall, the Heart Function Clinic experiences were seminal in my evolution from a physician concerned primarily with providing the best care for an individual patient to one who became increasingly aware of great gaps and opportunities for improvement in the care of whole populations of patients. Several things seemed to come together for me, such as an appreciation of the value of teamwork and partnership in care, an appreciation of a systematic and system approach to care, the power of measurements in answering old questions and asking new ones, and in driving improved practices and outcomes. It was an institution that seamlessly blended the academic and individual clinical attractions of medicine. In the blending they became more compelling to me than each was separately.

In short, the Heart Function Clinic became for me a crucible or practical laboratory for discovering and testing the principles of what I came to call health management.

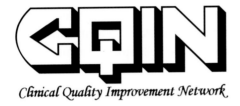

Figure 9.5: The logo of the Clinical Quality Improvement Network.

A third institution, the Clinical Quality Improvement Network, developed in the same time frame as EPICORE and the Heart Function Clinic. Its genesis was as follows.

As my colleagues and I at the University of Alberta were discovering the power of measurements in randomized clinical trials to improve care, others were, too. These physicians, nurses and related health professionals were also finding that measurements of usual daily practices were exposing care and outcome gaps. A number of these interested clinical stakeholders were meeting in common forums, particularly at scientific society gatherings and in steering committees to manage the increasing number of clinical trials in heart disease. We began to exchange thoughts and ideas on the care gaps, its causes and possible solutions.

One idea was to use some of the same network members and project principles, processes and data-gathering and analyses tools in the clinical trials and extend our pooled interest and resources to studies designed to test interventions to improve population effectiveness of therapy. So several centres came together to form CQIN, whose goals and objectives are outlined in Appendix C.

The idea to form a network for outcomes research and disease management was also practically stimulated by the serendipity of the first such study I was involved in that included data collection from more than one hospital

(Montague, Wong, Crowell et al. 1990). It was obvious, then, from the start, that cooperation was possible and it certainly facilitated more rapid collection of large population samples, practices and outcomes.

The project office and data-coordinating centre for the CQIN initiatives was the Epidemiology Coordinating and Research Centre (EPICORE) of the Division of Cardiology, University of Alberta, in Edmonton.

Beginning in the early 1990s, many CQIN projects were designed and implemented to measure and intervene upon usual practice patterns, particularly physicians' prescribing patterns, to improve practices and outcomes. The focus was predominantly heart disease, and the principal process used in the various projects was the standard combination of partnership and measurement.

The CQIN study targets were identified and agreed upon by the members, usually at meetings of all the partnership members and centres. Members and centres joined specific networks, however, according to their particular academic, clinical or geographic interests and the partnership members varied among the specific studies.

The governance model for CQIN was that of a steering committee of principal investigators representing the individual study centres, augmented by members of the project office and EPICORE. A representative example of the membership and infrastructure of a typical CQIN study is found in Appendix D.

A typical intervention tool—a physician order sheet designed to drive evidence-based practice and facilitate data collection—is reproduced in Appendix E.

Data sheets were carefully designed and tested to achieve the most accurate, precise and concise data abstraction for each study. The primary guideline in developing data sheets was that any data field must pass the test of "why." This meant we required a very good reason for retaining it in the final version of the data sheet. We had to be satisfied with the value the data was providing in contributing to answering the *a priori* question or questions that generated the study. That is, "It would be nice to have" was not a good enough reason to meet the selection criteria. This minimalist approach to data collection was adopted to avoid the trap of data mass, in which much time, effort and money can be expended in collecting, quality-assuring and collating data that are never interpreted or fed back.

Data sheets were backed up with detailed operating manuals and very specific data-coding keys to foster precise data collection. Data forms were filled out by trained data collectors for each patient in each centre, transferred to a computer disk and sent to the data centre at EPICORE for quality assurance, consolidation, analysis and feedback.

Periodic meetings of the members of CQIN were held, usually at six-month intervals. These member meetings were very important to the successful maintenance of the partnership and implementation of the various CQIN projects. They followed a standard format and agenda.

Basically, the meetings had two functions. The first was reporting the status of the research projects in progress, including feedback of data on patient recruitment, practices and outcomes and any issues or concerns with project progress. The second major purpose was to offer presentations by leading investigators and speakers on topics of practical current or possible future interest to the CQIN membership. This balance of feedback of latest study data and leading-edge education was a compellingly attractive combination for most members, providing an effective incentive for them to make the time and commitment required to travel to and participate in these meetings. In other words, the interests of the members were served and stimulated by the meetings. Along with a modest social event, usually held on the evening prior to the business portion of the meeting, these events held the membership's focus and stimulated performance during the relatively long duration of the CQIN studies.

The importance of the meetings as incentives to participate and contribute is all the more impressive because no one received a financial incentive for participating in the CQIN projects.

The funding for the projects was obtained from various sources, including medical research-granting agencies and industry. The principal costs incurred for a typical project were salary support for the data collectors and the expenses necessary for the steering committee meetings.

Over the last ten to fifteen years, a number of CQIN studies were mounted. Various specific targets in the general area of heart disease were studied, including practice patterns and outcomes for the acute ischemic syndromes of unstable angina and heart attack, as well as chronic disease states such as heart failure, atrial fibrillation and management of risk reduction for both high- and low-risk patients with the clinical manifestations of atherosclerosis. Results from these works are alluded to or illustrated in many of the figures in preceding chapters and are referenced in the bibliography.

CQIN was an innovative concept because it crystallized and helped to prove the feasibility of the partnership/measurement model of outcomes research and disease management. It showed the importance of measurements and communication in cementing and sustaining the partnerships over long periods. Experiences with interpreting the various study results broadened our minds and led to new concepts of what might become important players and institutions to lead and stimulate future improvements in health care. These experiences led us to explore other fields such as organizational behaviour, economics and health policy.

Overall, the results of the many studies of the CQIN group illustrated that there were many more similarities than differences in clinical practice patterns and care gaps, regardless of specific disease state, geography or physician type.

In short, CQIN confirmed the ubiquity of care gaps and the feasibility of using a patient management plan based on partnership and repeated measurement and feedback of practices and processes to inform the players and stimulate the closure of care gaps.

CQIN was a network of centres of excellence, or centres committed to measuring and intervening to become excellent in their practices and improve their outcomes. As it evolved, so did concepts and questions about a possible new model for active population health management or interventional epidemiology. Specifically, some of my colleagues began to wonder if it was possible to have a *province of excellence*, since health care policy and management in Canada is so closely related to and largely funded by the provinces.

I was one of the people who began to think that the centre of excellence model represented by CQIN, although great as a demonstration and proof of concept model, might not be good enough to actually improve practices and outcomes in a whole province. The question then became: could the ideas, recipes and processes proven feasible in CQIN be adapted for an entire Canadian health management entity, a Canadian health maintenance organization or a whole province?

As events unfolded, the answer became clear. It was yes. More specifically, it was ICONS, and ICONS became the icon.

Chapter 10

A PIVOTAL EXPERIENCE: IMPROVING CARDIOVASCULAR OUTCOMES IN NOVA SCOTIA (ICONS)

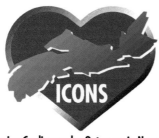

Improving Cardiovascular Outcomes in Nova Scotia

Figure 10.1: The logo of the ICONS partnership and project.

In late 1995 I began to consider seriously whether it would be possible to take some of the lessons learned from the experiences of CQIN, EPICORE and the Heart Function Clinic to develop a large-scale version of disease management. Specifically, I wondered if it was possible to mount a province-wide, partnership-measurement model of disease management for a major burden of illness.

At the same time, the large Canadian pharmaceutical company, Merck Frosst, was recognizing the importance of the gap between usual care and what best care could be. They understood that the undertreatment of many patients meant that no one—not patients, not providers, not payers—was obtaining the optimal health outcomes or social impact from the discovery and development of their and others' innovative products (see Figure 3.1). And they forecast that closure of care gaps, using evidence-based practices in a disease management model, might be a positive public health initiative, and also represent a successful business plan.

So I began discussions with Paul Howes, who was then the president of Merck Frosst, which ultimately led to my next career change. As a result of these talks, I moved to Montreal and joined Merck Frosst in early 1996. My major goals in making this change were to build a team within the company and develop external partnerships to evaluate the business and societal value of a practical and flexible partnership measurement model of disease management. This entailed demonstrating the model's feasibility in terms of acceptance by community stakeholders, academics and payers, as well as flexibility in its application across geographic and political boundaries and, ultimately, its sustainability and its transportability to various diseases and settings.

It is certainly gratifying, and some say vital, to begin a new endeavour with an early success to ensure long-term success. I guess it is fair to say, that in this regard, I got lucky. I got ICONS.

ICONS stands for Improving Cardiovascular Outcomes in Nova Scotia. In its original concept, ICONS was a five-year study to track the heart health of Nova Scotians (Cox, on behalf of the ICONS Investigators 1999). It was conceived as a province-wide, partnership-measurement model of disease management to focus on patients with both acute and chronic heart problems. More specifically, it was to evaluate the pre-hospital, in-hospital and post-hospital care of patients with heart attacks, unstable angina, congestive heart failure and atrial fibrillation. The goals included improvement in access to and processes of care, as well as eliminating any treatment biases and improving patient outcomes. It fostered optimal care as evidence-based, comprehensive and seamless, with the patient and his or her concerns as the central value.

ICONS was launched in 1997 and the proof of concept or initial research phase ended in 2002. Because of its very beneficial impact on the cardiovascular health of the population and its successful integration of community-based administrative culture and processes, ICONS became an operational program of the Department of Health of Nova Scotia in 2002.

In the view of health policy makers and others primarily concerned with administration of health care, this successful disease management initiative was a major innovation and achievement in organizational behaviour in primary health care (Montague, Cox, Kramer et al. 2003). And as we concluded in a summary overview written last year, the bottom-line recommendation remains: the ICONS model of partnership and measurement-driven management should be considered for other disease states and areas where the goals are closing care gaps and delivering the best health to the most people at the best cost.

Why Nova Scotia?

Why does Nova Scotia have such a significant impact on the Canadian scene? It can't be just their curlers, although as I write this chapter the Nova Scotia men's team has just won the 2004 Canadian championship. As you will recall, the current Canadian women's champion is also from Nova Scotia. Perhaps they are trying harder to do better?

In population health, Nova Scotia may have an outsized impact in part because it is relatively small. With a fairly stable and homogeneous population of about a million people living on a peninsula with one medical school and one large university hospital complex in Halifax with well-defined referral patterns, Nova Scotia forms a feasible, manageable living laboratory for outcomes research and disease management projects.

This natural advantage for interventional epidemiology was being supported in the mid-nineties by a visionary provincial government that had devised a strategic blueprint for health system improvement in 1994, followed by an information systems strategy in 1995 and a health business plan in 1998. Themes such as integration, accountability, outcomes research, evidence-based decision making and performance reporting featured consistently in these plans.

This holistic view of health was apparent at all levels of the Nova Scotia government during early information-sharing sessions with various players. A few stand out in my memory. One occurred during a meeting with Premier John Savage and Health Minister Bernard Boudreau. Premier Savage asked me what the pros and cons of ICONS over several years for Nova Scotia might be if we were to go ahead. In particular, he asked what Minister Boudreau might expect as upsides and downsides in his budget planning.

Based largely on my experience with initiatives like the Heart Function Clinic and the CQIN projects, I predicted that Minister Boudreau might see an increase in the use of efficacious medications and out-patient services, but a decrease in hospitalizations and an improvement in survival for the principal target diseases of heart attack, unstable angina and heart failure and a net benefit, both fiscally and clinically, for Nova Scotia. Premier Savage seemed willing to take this system view and he accepted these predictions with enough faith and courage to proceed in the partnership.

The other anecdote that succinctly illustrated the government's sense of the value of a system view of health care occurred during the ICONS launch events in early 1997, one of which was a press conference. A reporter posed a question to Minister Boudreau: "Why," he asked, "was Nova Scotia prepared to invest in the disease management partnership for heart diseases? What could be gained?" Minister Boudreau replied: "We are tired of managing by costs alone. We want to manage by outcomes."

At the time, I thought this was an extraordinary insight for a minister of health to recognize and verbalize. I certainly felt Florence Nightingale would have been very gratified to hear such expressions of value for measuring patient outcomes and using them to guide health policy.

In my continued experience with successive governments and health administrators in Nova Scotia over the relatively long time frame of ICONS, these impressions of vision and out-of-the-box thinking that permeated health care policy did not change.

There were other compelling reasons to consider a program to improve the heart health of Nova Scotians in the mid- and late nineties. In Canada at that time, Nova Scotians had the second highest rate of cardiovascular deaths, the third lowest life expectancy and the highest number of people in surveys who reported only fair or poor health. Nova Scotia had also just completed and published in 1996 the results of an outcomes analysis of patients with heart attacks in the province. This project confirmed the high burden of heart disease in Nova Scotia, and it also demonstrated the feasibility and the power of many partners and health centres working together.

And at that time as well, national surveys of citizens' perception of the quality of our health care had for the first time shown that more people thought our health care was fair or poor, compared to excellent or very good. All in all, it was a good time for a significant effort to make things better.

The ICONS Partnership

ICONS was a partnership of government, academia, community health stakeholders—including doctors, nurses, pharmacists and patients—and business.

An inclusive list of the members of ICONS and their affiliations is provided in Appendix F.

At its core was the steering committee, made up of a clinical team from each of the major health districts of Nova Scotia (see Figure 10.2).

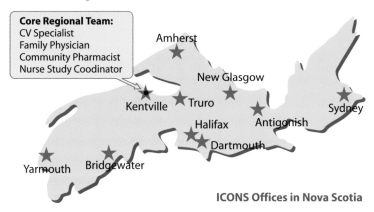

Core Regional Team:
CV Specialist
Family Physician
Community Pharmacist
Nurse Study Coodinator

Amherst

New Glasgow

Kentville   Truro

Halifax   Antigonish

Sydney

Dartmouth

Yarmouth   Bridgewater

ICONS Offices in Nova Scotia

Figure 10.2: Geographic location of the regional teams composing the community-based clinical leadership for the ICONS project. Each team consisted of a cardiovascular specialist, an internist or cardiologist, a family physician, a community pharmacist and a nurse coordinator: the community face of ICONS working across traditional functional and geographic borders. Adapted, with permission, from ICONS.

In the context of the culture of ICONS, it is fair to say the government partner expected ICONS to develop a system-wide evaluation of care and outcomes and possibly link them. ICONS also provided an experiment in examining and improving performance that, if successful, might be expanded to other conditions. ICONS offered the capability to support evidence-based clinical decision making and some promise of further developing information technology and communications among partners to advance care.

I felt that the other steering committee members had mixed expectations. The academic members recognized the opportunity for Nova Scotia to have an advantage in being at the leading edge of population health research or interventional epidemiology. Community-based stakeholders—including physicians, pharmacists and patients—viewed membership in ICONS as innovative. It was innovative because public-private partnerships in health care were new and somewhat in vogue as a concept worthy of testing. It was innovative as well because it provided an opportunity for many of these stakeholders to contribute to the generation and dissemination of important medical information that might lead to equally important medical decisions for the whole province. Although they may not have been asked to make such a contribution before, nonetheless, they recognized the opportunity to contribute, and it was the first step in setting up a province-wide Hawthorne Effect.

All members probably viewed the partnership and project goals as manageable and attainable, but I suspect that if everyone had known how difficult it would be to build and maintain the partnership, they may have had second thoughts about joining. In particular, I think the value and difficulty of communications were probably underestimated. One of the regional leaders was Dr. Ron Hatheway, a cardiologist in Bridgewater, Nova Scotia. Dr. Hatheway had been a former colleague and student of mine during his residency training at Halifax's Victoria General Hospital.

One of my clearest memories of working with Ron was of an evening when he was the senior resident and I was the staff cardiologist on call for the hospital. We had just recently agreed on a hospital protocol for administering clot-busting therapy to patients with acute heart attacks. But no one had actually administered these drugs to a patient when Ron called me that Saturday evening. The patient Ron called me about was a young woman, who was still of child-bearing age. Ron thought she should receive the clot buster to minimize her heart damage, but he was exercising due diligence in assessing the risks and benefits of the therapy, which was new at the time. He wanted to be certain that he was recommending a therapy that would result in more benefit than harm. I concurred with Ron, we administered the new therapy and the patient did very well.

Ron Hatheway's commitment to optimal patient care and his courage in pursuing his commitment, including the courage to go first, was significant.

Perhaps Ron felt he was exercising an equivalent prudent risk taking once again when he accepted an invitation to join the steering committee of ICONS. I don't know because I never asked him, but perhaps I should have. However, one thing I did ask Ron, in the context of a meeting we organized in Montreal to share some of the emerging best practices from ICONS, was to summarize the major practical initiatives he felt were critical to get ICONS up and running in the South Shore region of Nova Scotia.

Figure 10.3 is Ron Hatheway's. It represents a fair summary of what it took to build the partnership of ICONS across the province. It represents the product of on-the-job experience and training, learning from a starting point of expediency and goodwill.

None of it was I able to predict or suggest before ICONS was implemented. In the great scheme of things, it is a prime example of the teacher becoming the student.

Building the Partnership
Communicate, Communicate, Communicate
- Regional office set-up
- Letter of introduction from Minister of Health
- Letter from local hospital CEO to all local sites
- Liaisons with hospital departments
- Implementation of on-line database
- Multi-disciplinary in-services at all sites
- Physician CME and office visits
- Promotional materials at all sites
- Pharmacy visits
- Public launch—reception and press conference
- Media contracts

Figure 10.3: Summary of communication and relational marketing efforts in the Bridgewater region of Nova Scotia to mount and initially ground the ICONS partnership. Adapted, with permission, from personal communication with R. Hatheway.

Sustaining the partnership was also important, considering the duration of the first phase of ICONS lasted more than five years. Several interventions were utilized during ICONS's long research phase. They included professional stakeholder and patient education, use of facile care maps and practice guidelines, physician prompts and benchmarking of practices and outcomes (see Figure 10.4 and Appendices G, H, I and J).

Above all other interventions, however, the most important was measurement and feedback of the relevant-to-stakeholders clinical data gathered in ICONS. This brings to mind a very appropriate thought that sums up the value of this most important intervention for effective health management partnerships. Although the statement was not made in primary reference to health care partnerships, it certainly has occurred to me many times and I suspect it would also have Florence Nightingale nodding her head. It is from a Harvard University educator, Charles Deutsch. Of partnerships, he said: "We talk about them as if they were exhilarating, but they are usually exhausting and sometimes maddening. They have to focus relentlessly on results or they are likely to get lost attending to process" (Montague 2000).

Measurements facilitate buy-in and stimulate the next iteration of the Hawthorne Effect. Without measurement, partners risk a non-productive focus on the process and politics of forming and operating a partnership. With measurement in place, you have the motivation to do more, better.

Sustaining the Partnership

Measure, Inform

■ **Interventions**
- Measurement and feedback
- Patient and provider newsletters
- Physician workshops
- Care maps, algorithms, discharge forms
- Patient education
- Pharmacy monitoring, compliance programs
- Web site (www.icons.ns.ca)

■ **Benchmarking**

Figure 10.4: Summary of interventions in all regions of Nova Scotia to sustain and advance the ICONS partnership and its goals of improving cardiovascular outcomes in the province. Adapted, with permission, from ICONS.

I have another vivid memory of the ICONS partnership. Some of the ICONS members have called it the "magic" of ICONS. I observed it during a steering committee meeting about midway through the research phase of ICONS. It was a Sunday morning and we were in a Halifax hotel. The participants in the meeting were a subgroup of the steering committee responsible for evaluating possible substudies for ICONS. I sat beside Joan Fraser, the executive director of the Heart and Stroke Foundation of Nova Scotia. Mrs. Fraser had been an early proponent of ICONS and an original member of the steering committee. Previously, I had met Mrs. Fraser when I lived in Halifax. At that time, Mrs. Fraser was not formally involved in health care, but she definitely had a sense of civic responsibility; she was a citizenship court judge.

I knew that Mrs. Fraser, like all members of the steering committee, was not receiving any remuneration for working on ICONS on a beautiful Sunday in the spring. I also knew she usually attended church on Sundays. Yet, here she was in a room without windows, actively participating in the debate about what might be the best substudy to support the overall ICONS project. I was impressed and interested enough to ask her why she was there, as opposed to in church or home with her family. Mrs. Fraser replied very simply: "But Terry, this is important."

I had the impression she felt it was probably an unnecessary question on my part. That is, for her, she was compellingly and obviously doing important work, and I think she assumed that would be obvious to any person involved in health care. I recognized this from a scientific point of view, but what Mrs. Fraser added to my appreciation was a visceral understanding that it was important also because people like her thought it was very important from a community point of view. It assured me of the moral authority of this type of health management. Partnership grounded in the community is attractive to the members of the community, and they willingly contribute because they understand how important it is.

Mrs. Fraser also provided me with another very important insight. It occurred during a dinner meeting as part of a larger gathering of members of several disease management projects designed to share best practices. She was part of a conversation with Dr. David Johnstone and me. The discussion focused on the rapid and large enrolment of patients in the ICONS project during the first year. Dr. Johnstone and I recognized that the several thousand patients who signed up in a year represented an exceptionally positive accomplishment in a clinical research project. In fact, slower than expected enrolment is often a big worry for people overseeing a clinical trial. It certainly was a concern during the SOLVD trial, in which we had both taken part, and it was also a problem in the SCAT trial.

As I remember it, Dr. Johnstone and I were more or less assuming credit for ICONS's incredible enrolment statistics. We thought we had gotten something right in the study's design and implementation, right from the start. We were thinking of something along the lines of a compellingly attractive protocol or charismatic regional medical leaders. In fact, I still think both of these factors were operative in ICONS. However, Mrs. Fraser suggested another reason that, over time, I have come to believe was likely a greater contributor to the exceptional patient acceptance of ICONS than any academic or charismatic medical factors. Mrs. Fraser's contention was that ICONS's patient acceptance was high because everyone associated with the Heart and Stroke Foundation, from its executive director to its thousands of volunteers in Nova Scotia, was firmly behind the ICONS goals and they told patients and families that ICONS was a worthwhile project and should be supported.

In other words, it was a matter of trust. Patients trusted and listened to people they knew and respected in their community. I have come to think of this trust as a social kin to the health belief theories of medical decision making in which patients accept or reject provider advice on specific therapies. Patients may also have a variety of beliefs with regard to their support or participation in health research. Using two-way communication and community-grounded, trusted individuals or institutions to aid in the communication is important for vital project functions such as recruitment.

Mrs. Fraser was not the only steering committee member who impressed me with her community orientation and contributions. One of the ICONS substudy protocols originated from the ideas of a community pharmacist who practised in a very small town in northeastern Nova Scotia. His presentation, with the design of a randomized clinical trial, was compelling, was accepted and ultimately carried out. In subsequent committee meetings of the partnership, as well as in the meet-and-greet activities, I noticed how influential and respected this pharmacist was in his dealings with other members of ICONS. This steering committee member epitomized for me the invisible and largely untapped community-based talent, someone who valued population health science and civic sensitivity, the type of professional who was likely available in any community. He was a practical manifestation of the moral authority inherent in the community. It just needs tapping and perhaps some measurement to make it operational.

The ICONS Measurements and Results

Many variables were measured in the ICONS project. They included demographic and clinical data on who was incurring cardiac disease, being admitted and investigated in hospitals, who was being treated, who was surviving, being discharged and followed up in the communities of Nova Scotia (Cox, on behalf of the ICONS Investigators 1999). Rates of use of evidence-based therapies were a primary measure for ICONS's research purposes. The project team was aiming for a 25 percent increase in the use of proven therapies for each of the major disease states being targeted: heart attack, unstable angina and the abnormal heart electrical rhythm, atrial fibrillation (Cox, on behalf of the ICONS Investigators 1999).

It was also expected that regional variations in care patterns and access to services, as well as predictors of differences in therapy use, would be possible over the course of the study.

As of 2003, more than 60,000 hospital admissions or community referrals for the target disease states had been assessed, involving about 35,000 separate patients (Montague, Cox, Kramer et al. 2003). The following are some of ICONS's positive results.

Who Is Hospitalized with Heart Disease?

Of the almost 9,000 patients admitted to thirty-two Nova Scotia hospitals with heart attacks between 1997 and 2002, 62 percent were male and 38 percent were female. Fifteen percent of the males were older than eighty years of age, but twice as many female heart attack patients were older than eighty.

For heart failure, the equivalent data were more than 12,000 admissions during the same time frame and 52 percent were female. The majority of these female heart failure patients (about 51 percent) were older than eighty years of age, compared to only 34 percent of the male patients with heart failure.

The bottom-line message here is that acute and chronic heart diseases are becoming or already are diseases of older women. As indicated in Figure 7.7, there is an accompanying social gap of older female heart patients, compared to men. Not only are the female patients older, they are poorer and more of them live alone.

How Were Patients Treated?

ICONS's primary goal was to determine whether a population-based patient health initiative would be associated with a 25 percent increase in the use of proven index therapies in the target diseases over the proposed five-year research phase of the project (Cox, on behalf of the ICONS Investigators 1999).

The trends in prescription patterns for the index drugs suggest that the goal was largely achieved. Based on measurements between 1997 and 2001, in the first four years of ICONS, the use of angiotensin-converting enzyme inhibitors among heart failure patients rose from 47 percent to 67 percent at the time of discharge; the use of lipid-lowering statin drugs in heart attack patients increased from 30 percent to 58 percent; and the use of anti-coagulant therapy for preventing strokes in patients with atrial fibrillation rose from 47 percent to 61 percent.

In fact, there was a general and continuous increase in all proven therapies in the target diseases. For example, in the treatment of heart failure, the use of beta-blocker drugs increased from about 40 percent to nearly 70 percent among the hospital patient population. And the similarly changed pattern for heart attack prescriptions is illustrated in Figure 10.5.

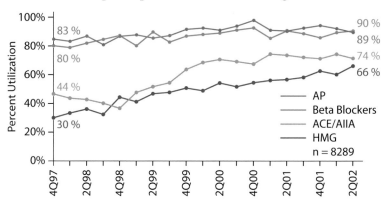

Figure 10.5: Increased use of proven medical therapies at discharge among 8,289 patients with heart attack, or acute myocardial infarction, admitted to Nova Scotia hospitals between 1997 and 2002. AP = anti-platelet therapy; ACE/AIIA = angiotensin-converting enzyme inhibitors/angiotensin-receptor antagonists; HMG = lipid-lowering statin medications; Q = quarter of a year. Reproduced, with permission, from *Hospital Quarterly* (Montague, Cox, Kramer et al. 2003).

There was an accompanying decrease in the use of non-proven therapies in some diseases. For example, in the hospital management of heart failure, the use of digitalis drugs decreased from 38 percent in 1997 to 27 percent in 2001.

In benchmark terms, I believe these practice patterns are the best practices that have yet been reported for any large patient population. In the heart attack group, the practice patterns by 2002 could even be said to be nearing theoretically ideal goals. But things can always be better.

When I look at Figure 10.5, one thing that strikes me every time is that the levels of use for the older drugs are truly remarkable, particularly the use of beta blockers (90 percent). I remember some of the doctors' comments fifteen years ago when we first began to measure the use of these drugs at about the 25–30 percent level. Some doctors said that was the proper population level of use; they couldn't be safely used in any more patients. Well, the Nova Scotia data suggest that the lowball opinion was not true.

An extrapolation of this thinking to the newer drug therapies, such as the statins and angiotensin-converting enzyme inhibitors, is that their current use levels are still too low, even in Nova Scotia. They, too, can reach use levels of greater than 90 percent, I believe. If they do, they will further improve important outcomes such as increased survival and reduced rehospitalization.

What Were the Patient Outcomes?

Things have gotten better. In terms of survival, the overall in-hospital death rate among heart attack patients fell from over 16 percent in 1997 and 1998 to slightly under 13 percent in 2000 and 2001. As in the previous CQIN experience, the greatest decrease in risk of dying occurred in older patients. For patients younger than seventy-five years of age, the death rate decreased from 8.4 percent to 6.7 percent. In patients older than seventy-five, on the other hand, the risk of dying fell from about 30 percent in the early days of ICONS to about 24 percent in 2000 and 2001. And also as in the previous CQIN experience, this greater impact in improving survival was attained despite less use of proven therapy in older ICONS patients (see Figure 4.2).

157

In terms of rehospitalization for patients with heart attack, the data show that patients treated in 1997 and 1998 had a readmission rate of about 41 percent one year after their initial discharge. In comparison, ICONS heart attack patients treated in 1999 and 2000 had a risk for readmission of only 35 percent in the year following their initial admission, a significant improvement in this important clinical and fiscal marker and outcome.

There were similar directional improvements in the risk of dying and readmission for heart failure patients, but they were of a lesser degree. For example, the risk of dying in hospital with heart failure decreased from 15 percent to 14 percent between 1997/1998 and 2000/2001. The risk of readmission for these patients in the same time frame decreased from 40 percent to 38 percent. These heart failure patients are obviously not only older but sicker. Things can be better.

Transition of ICONS

ICONS has become an icon in Canadian population health and disease management.

In its first phase, the ICONS project defined some paths for others to follow, including the value of a dedicated collegial governance structure, careful planning and discussion of process and measurements, adequate resources, interpartner respect and sensitivity. It developed innovative tools beyond the originally conceived measurements, including standardized care maps (see Appendices G and H) and discharge orders (see Appendix I) to facilitate comprehensiveness and seamlessness of care from hospital to the community.

ICONS markedly advanced techniques to enhance provider and patient communication, education and buy-in, all of which likely contributed to the very positive Hawthorne Effect, along with the measurement and feedback process, in encouraging improved practices and outcomes. An example of the stakeholder newsletter used in ICONS is in Appendix J.

ICONS brought a culture of measurement to evidence-based practices and multidisciplinary health management. It enhanced interregional goodwill and sharing of best practices, and it laid the framework for a provincial cardiac program that was part of the day-to day-strategy and function of the Department of Health.

To become fully operational and ensure long-term success, ICONS must now benchmark against important factors for the Department of Health. They include administrative integration with other existing structures such as the regional health authorities, persistent community orientation, accountability and sustainability. Most of these governmental benchmarks had already been built into the original ICONS design, particularly community focus and accountability through measurement. Sustainability, however, did not perhaps receive proper consideration in the first phase of ICONS and some catch-up had to be done.

As I observed ICONS evolve over the last several years, it was obvious to me that the leadership of two people in particular was critical to its success.

First was the academic leadership provided by Dr. Jafna Cox, a young cardiologist and epidemiologist who led the robust scientific underpinnings of the design, implementation and interpretation of the continuous body of knowledge generated by this unique public health endeavour.

Second was the role played by the chair, Dr. David Johnstone, a gifted clinical cardiologist and academic physician. He has a sense of community altruism that extends beyond even Nova Scotia. Currently, he is president of the Canadian Cardiovascular Society, the main professional organization of Canada's providers of heart care. He can and does take both the individual and the broad population view of health care. Moreover, he does it with competence and grace.

Keeping a team as diverse as ICONS's steering committee focused and pulling in the same direction for several years definitely meets General Schwarzkopf's definition of leadership. Dr. Johnstone led people where they might otherwise not have gone. He also led them where people had never gone before, at least in our country.

I think this experience gives him a unique view of contemporary and perhaps future health management strategy for Canada. Dr. Johnstone says the following:

> Finding the optimal balance in quality, cost and access is a formidable challenge in health care. For effective patient health management, you need an accurate snapshot of what you are currently doing (data collection), a dedicated team of experts to interpret the data and translate the findings (health service researchers) and a committed body of stakeholders that have a common purpose of ensuring that individual patients receive the best care possible at an affordable cost.
>
> ICONS was successful because we had all the right ingredients and all the necessary players at the table. The magic of ICONS was that individuals and groups were encouraged to find solutions and believe in the process.
>
> One of our key success stories in the ICONS experience was the development of a network of Heart Function Clinics in Nova Scotia. Heart failure in Nova Scotia, like the rest of Canada, affects elderly patients and carries a very poor prognosis with a high mortality rate, need for rehospitalization and poor quality of life. Patients receive numerous medications, which all have the potential to interact in a negative manner. Many patients are required to take upwards of ten different medications a day, all with the potential to cause side effects and, in some cases, life-threatening situations.

Dr. Jafna Cox, the ICONS scientific director, presented baseline data to the steering committee and outlined a series of options, which could lessen the burden of these patients. One of the inescapable conclusions was that we had to do things differently. We encouraged the start-up of Heart Function Clinics, which were designed to provide patients with detailed understanding of their condition, how to take their medications, how to recognize worsening symptoms, how to shop for foods that are safe and, perhaps most importantly, how best to participate in the management of their underlying condition.

We found that Heart Function Clinics not only work in terms of decreasing mortality and readmission to hospital rates. Patients report improved satisfaction with their care and had an improved quality of life. We now are embarking on a program to increase the involvement of pharmacists as well as family doctors in the overall heart function team approach to this terrible condition. In an effort to decrease the travel burden involved with coming to the Heart Function Clinic, we are also developing a demonstration project to use tele-homecare as an adjunct to the Heart Function Clinic. We hope that telehomecare can be used to help reinforce many of the educational components of the clinic as well as to monitor basic clinical data such as weight, blood pressure and symptomatic status.

Many other valuable ideas which have been acted upon came from our regional members of the ICONS steering committee. They continuously challenge us to get the right people at the table, give them the best information possible and sit back and listen closely.

As we go forward together, I am increasingly convinced this community base is the cornerstone of our future.

A Closing ICONS Lesson

As one considers the processes involved in the components of total, comprehensive and seamless care, and realizes the increasing empowerment from new information management systems, attributing exclusivity of ownership or responsibility to any single group to improve imperfect diagnosis, prescription, compliance and access seems simplistic.

With gains in knowledge, there is an associated increased sense of comfort for one stakeholder group to comment on or work within the traditional fiefdoms of other groups to design and effect solutions to the care gap.

In summary, there is much accountability and opportunity to share.

For example, in the ICONS project, over time, patient members of the steering committee gained experience in issues such as the provincial burden of illness of congestive heart failure. As well, the gaps in contemporary care and associated opportunities for improved care were visible. With this enhanced knowledge and experience, patients and patient advocacy groups felt empowered and compelled to express their opinion to the politicians and health policy decision makers as to how to best improve future access to care for the affected patients.

In a very practical way, the patients felt they had the responsibility to give the government their opinion, based on their new medical knowledge and experience, combined with their long-term knowledge of local social and political currents. And so they did. They weighed in with advice on proposals such as the value of heart function clinics, and where they should be located to obtain best effect for the most people.

When I first realized this empowering impact on patients who were intimately involved in population health partnerships, I was surprised. The phenomenon was not an *a priori* goal of ICONS. Nonetheless, I have come to recognize the value of this level of patient involvement in health care discussions and strategic decisions. We are doing the right thing when we put patients first, as the title of this book suggests, and we are giving patients, with their aspirations and their concerns, the primacy of position in the health care debate that they merit. Their perceptions are very important and to ignore them or undervalue them is to risk doing our health system a great disservice.

But perception is reality only to a degree. The survey data, outlined in Figure 3.4, suggest a need to broaden the knowledge and perceptions of patients. Even in an ideal "Patients First" world it is necessary to consider that quality in health care and outcomes means more than closing gaps in access to diagnostic and therapeutic services. I agree with Durhane Wong-Reiger that if patients had more of the available knowledge regarding care gaps, the cost of closing them and the cost of not closing them, their contributions to the debate on how to balance the principal driving forces of access, quality and costs would markedly improve the policy decision-making process.

The challenge involves how to do this well. ICONS provided great value in identifying the opportunity and illuminating the initial path. It remains for subsequent partnerships and projects to further advance the cause. Things can be better.

Chapter 11

OTHER EXPERIENCES IN
PATIENT HEALTH MANAGEMENT

At the time the Patient Health team was created at Merck Frosst, I felt that health care in Canada was at a crossroads.

The restructuring phase of health management, with its focus on cost reduction through restricted access to products and services, was still evolving and growing. The merits of restrictive policy actions included an aura of administrative simplicity, with rapid implementation and likelihood of obtaining the desired money goal in the component budget being targeted, for example, reducing expenditures on a specific drug or drug class. On the other hand, there was a body of evidence suggesting that payer-centred, restricted-access health policies produced offsetting, unintended, but adverse, clinical and economic outcomes and unsatisfied patients and providers.

Consequently, I felt it was important to develop some feasible options to single-component, restricted-access health policy. My colleagues and I proposed patient health management as one promising alternative (Montague, Sidel, Erhardt et al. 1997). We envisioned the major advantages of this alternative strategy to include evidence-based, patient-centred and seamless care. The major disadvantages were the long-term commitment to partnership building and to the measurement and education required to assess the power of this approach in making best care the usual care in an accountable way.

As we were characterizing these options, ICONS was just being launched.

We anticipated ICONS's likelihood of success in part because of fairly extensive previous experience in managing various heart diseases with the CQIN teams. However, we also recognized the skepticism of many observers and players in the Canadian health arena toward the partnership/measurement model of disease management that we were proposing. In particular, we recognized that the lack of experience with diseases other than heart disease was contributing to the skepticism.

Since that time in 1997, we have engaged in many other disease management—or patient health management—partnerships in different diseases and in various provinces. Several of these initiatives are graphically depicted in Figure 11.1.

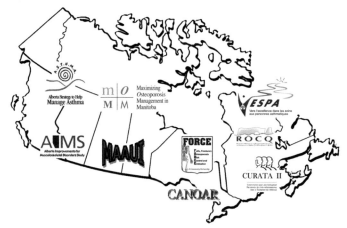

Figure 11.1: Geographic and iconic representation of ongoing disease-management projects in which the Patient Health team at Merck Frosst has contributed to the partnerships. The project logos represent, from West to East: Alberta Study to Help Manage Asthma (ASTHMA); Alberta Improvements for Musculoskeletal Disorders Study (AIMS); Maximizing Osteoporosis Management in Manitoba (MOMM); Manitoba Anti-inflammatory Appropriate Utilization Initiative (MAAUI); Falls, Fracture and Osteoporosis Risk Control and Evaluation (FORCE) project; Canadian Osteoarthritis Rx (CANOAR) program; Vers l'excellence dans les soins aux personnes asthmatiques (VESPA); Recognizing Osteoporosis and its Consequences in Quebec (ROCQ) and Concertation pour une Utilisation Raisonnée des Anti-inflammatoires dans le Traitement de l'Arthrose (CURATA).

The diseases covered by the programs shown in Figure 11.1 include asthma, arthritis and other inflammatory diseases that require therapy to control inflammation and pain, and osteoporosis. In addition to these projects, which, like ICONS, are pan-provincial in scope, our Patient Health group has been involved in several other developmental projects involving the management of patients with migraine, childhood asthma, depression, kidney disease and diabetes.

While there are differences in the design features of these disease management projects, they all operate with the mantra that things can be better and they all use some variant of the partnership/measurement recipe in their structures and processes. It may be helpful to describe a few of the projects in more detail to provide a better feeling for variations and similarities in contemporary Canadian disease management programs and partnerships.

Alberta Strategy to Help Manage Asthma (ASTHMA)

It is theoretically possible to mount a patient-health management program to help improve care and outcomes for any disease. It seems reasonable, however, at least in the formative years of patient health management, to focus limited resources on diseases that are a big burden for our society. In such a situation, where the target population is large, even small improvements in prescribing or compliance patterns can bring large public health and economic gains.

Asthma is such a disease. It affects 5 to 10 percent of the population and is an enormous family and economic burden because of its high prevalence and frequent exacerbations, which are often associated with time lost from school and work. The ASTHMA project in Alberta developed out of the recognition of the growing burden of illness and the care gap relating to asthma.

The partnership is composed of approximately 180 community physicians from across the province, academic specialists in respiratory disease from the universities of Calgary and Alberta, the Alberta Medical Association and the Alberta Family Practice Research Network, patients and their advocacy groups, including the Alberta Lung Association, government (Alberta Health and Wellness) and industry (Merck Frosst). The principal governance structures are the executive and steering committees and the EPICORE centre is the data-management facility for the project (Sharpe et al. 2004).

The project was planned in three phases: (1) a measurement of current management practices and identification of care gaps, (2) sequential feedback and (3) remeasurement and refeedback of practices as they are modified by the project interventions, with insights determined from the measurements and focus-group analyses.

The findings from the initial ASTHMA measurements are now being fed back to the stakeholders (Tsuyuki, Sin, Sharpe et al. 2004). Briefly, these early data revealed that more than half of the patients were unlikely to receive any form of education about asthma treatment and were equally unlikely to be using spirometry measurements to verify diagnosis, confirm severity and guide treatment. Only 2 percent were following a written action plan for treatment. A patient survey revealed that self-management was infrequent and the overall control of symptoms and care was essentially unchanged from five years previously, despite publication and dissemination of practice guidelines and expert reports. So, things can be better.

In future measurements I anticipate we will see practices improve as the ASTHMA partnership is stimulated by their own practice data and is able to benchmark those measurements against best, evidence-based practices.

Vers l'excellence dans les soins aux personnes asthmatiques (VESPA)

VESPA or TEAM (Towards Excellence in Asthma Management) is a broad-based, disease management partnership to improve asthma management in Quebec (Boulet et al. 2002). The academic leadership comes from pediatric and adult asthma specialists from Université Laval, Université de Montréal and McGill University. The other major institutional players include the Quebec Asthma Education Network, the Ministry of Health, the regional health authorities, the Fonds de Recherche en Santé du Québec (FRSQ), Santé Publique and several industry partners.

The advisory board membership for VESPA includes representation from the College of Physicians, Fédération des médecins omnipraticiens du Québec (FMOQ), community and academic pharmacists, nurses and respiratory therapists, as well as patients' associations such as Asthmedia, Quebec Lung Association and Asthma Allergy Information Association.

The principal goals of VESPA are reduction of the level of morbidity and improvement in the quality of life for asthmatic patients and optimization of the use of health care resources while improving the clinical management of asthma, including the promotion of self-management by asthmatics.

VESPA was designed in four phases:

• Phase I is a cartographic analysis of the distribution of asthma and its severity (see Figure 11.2).
• Phase II is a cohort baseline study of current patterns of prescribing practice and substudies of patient compliance and communication between patients and physicians.
• Phase III involves the first intervention, including initial feedback of measurements.
• Phase IV involves subsequent interventions and broadening of the partnership.

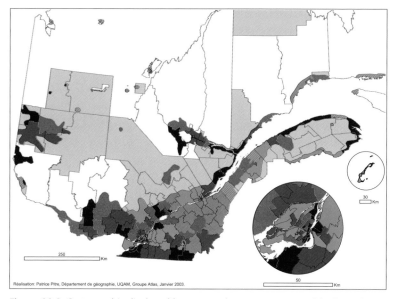

Réalisation: Patrice Pitre, Département de géographie, UQAM, Groupe Atlas, Janvier 2003.

Figure 11.2: Cartographic display of frequency of emergency room visits for patients from five to forty-four years of age with asthma in Quebec in 2000. Navy represents areas of higher incidence of visits; blue and white represent low-incidence areas; other colours fall within this spectrum. Reproduced, with permission, from VESPA. (Laurier, Blais, Kennedy et al. 2004.) Surveillance épidémiologique de l'asthme au Québec et variations régionales, 1999-2001: une analyse des banques de données.

The cartography study of VESPA has produced an accurate overview of the regional burden of this illness in the province. It has allowed an evidence-based focus for targeted interventions. For example, high-morbidity target regions for future interventions are Montreal, the Saguenay region and the region of Lac St-Jean. Quebec City, on the other hand, is a low-morbidity area, while the South Shore of Montreal, the City of Laval and the Eastern Townships are areas with a medium burden of illness. A second cartography study, covering the years 1999–2001, has been conducted to monitor the geographic evolution of asthma morbidity within the province (see Figure 11.2).

In Phase II, the specific goals were to define asthma case-management processes, including patient compliance and to compare the determinants of care gaps in high-morbidity regions versus low-morbidity regions. Major findings of the cohort study included significant gaps in communication and understanding between physicians and their patients in terms of perception of the severity of the disease, its symptomatic control and treatment action plans. For example, patients see themselves as less sick than their doctors see them.

In Phase III, the first wave of interventions included evaluation of an educational intervention targeted for the emergency room management team in caring for attacks in children aged one to fourteen, development of a tool to facilitate the patient-doctor consultation process in the physicians' office, assessment of spirometry use and its role in promoting attendance at asthma education centres in the community care setting and optimizing acute treatment at emergency rooms and referral to education centres for adult patients in high-morbidity regions.

A second wave of interventions in Phase III included development of a patient and family decision support process to facilitate understanding and removal of the causative role of domestic animals in asthma exacerbations, evaluation of an educational program (staffed by nurses), providing a hotline information and counselling service for all asthma patients in the moderate- and high-prevalence areas, and an assessment of the impact of a pharmacist education program on patients' use of medications.

The results of these interventions are currently being evaluated and planning is advancing for launch of Phase IV, in partnership with the FRSQ, using an innovative request for proposals from any interested groups in Quebec who feel they might benefit from association with the existing VESPA partnership and resources.

Four interventional projects have so far been accepted for further evaluation. They include innovative new areas of investigation, particularly focusing on care gaps not addressed during Phase III. One highlight is assessment of integrated care programs, including those using facile electronic devices to monitor patient compliance and safety and enhance physicians' prescribing decisions. All of these peer-reviewed intervention protocols include outcome measures of patient morbidity and quality of care.

Another highlight of Phase IV is the creation of an alliance between the Faculties of Medicine of the Université de Montréal and Université Laval for the specific purpose of developing a provincial asthma education program for health professionals. The impact on morbidity and medical practice of this program will be evaluated as well.

My sense of the increasing importance of VESPA is that its vitality and robustness in study goals and their measurement, along with its ever-broadening community partnerships, will lead to its strategic evolution and sustainability as a provincial asthma program for both pediatric and adult patients.

Maximizing Osteoporosis Management in Manitoba (MOMM)

Osteoporosis is a disease of older people, particularly older postmenopausal women, in which there is gradual demineralization of bones. This age-related decrease in bone minerals, with probably some additional contribution from altered bone structure or architecture, puts those who have it at increased risk of breaking bones important to their stature and their ability to walk, bones such as those in the spine or hip.

The Maximizing Osteoporosis Management in Manitoba (MOMM) project was initiated in 2000, driven by the belief of many people working in the area of women's health care that osteoporosis is a disease of significant risk to older women and that it is very much under-recognized, underdiagnosed and undertreated in our society.

MOMM is composed of Manitoba Health, the University of Manitoba, the Manitoba Clinic and Merck Frosst, with support and endorsement from the Manitoba Chapter of the Osteoporosis Society of Canada, the Manitoba Pharmaceutical

Association and the Society of Obstetricians and Gynecologists of Canada. Briefly, the mission of the broad MOMM coalition of government, academic and primary care providers, health care industry and patient advocacy partners is to optimize osteoporosis care and outcomes throughout Manitoba.

The specific objectives include determining the prevalence of women with osteoporosis who are at increased risk for fracture and the care they receive, anticipating care gaps and improving the use of evidence-based prevention and treatment strategies through targeted interventions, assessing changes in practice following intervention(s), including assessing the impact of MOMM on disease awareness, patient diagnosis and treatment patterns.

One unique feature of the MOMM project is its use of different and complementary sources of data, including direct surveys of Manitoba women over fifty to assess their risk of osteoporosis and fracture, as well as a survey of diagnostic use of bone mineral density (BMD) testing data from the working clinics where this test is located, and analyses of existing and linked databases maintained by Manitoba Health, including the Drug Program Information Network, the Research Registry, the Manitoba Health Physician Registry and the Medical Claims and Hospital files. This MOMM advantage is due to the robust databases previously constructed by Manitoba Health and the academic community, and their commitment to using them to facilitate outcomes research in the province.

MOMM is still in progress, but the preliminary findings of the study thus far suggest that osteoporosis is a significant public health problem for Manitoba. Results indicate that one in two women in Manitoba over fifty may be at significantly increased risk for fractures. And, as shown in Figure 4.5, there is a very large care gap between optimal diagnosis and treatment and the usual practices for women at high risk. In 2001–2002 only 20 percent of the highest risk patients with previous spine or hip fractures were receiving appropriate diagnostic testing or proven medical therapy to reduce their risk for future fracture. Things can be better.

Interventions to broaden the community provider partnership and introduce interventions to increase recognition of high-risk patients are currently underway. Things will be better.

Falls, Fracture and Osteoporosis Risk Control and Evaluation (FORCE)

FORCE stands for the Falls, Fracture and Osteoporosis Risk Control and Evaluation project. It is a coalition of community, government and industry partners working toward a goal of reducing osteoporosis-related complications in Northern Ontario, centred in Sault Ste. Marie. The partners include the Group Health Centre, the Algoma Health Unit, Sault Area hospital, the Algoma Community Care Access Centre and several pharmaceutical companies—Aventis Pharma, Procter & Gamble Canada, Lilly Canada and Merck Frosst.

The background and rationale for FORCE stem from several factors, in particular a growing awareness of the large numbers of older people in the general population, and that falls and fractures in this group account for a significant proportion of the community's total morbidity. For example, more women may die as a result of osteoporotic fractures each year than from breast and ovarian cancer combined.

FORCE's principal assumption is that effective coordination and application of available community resources in Sault Ste. Marie—for example, a multidisciplinary assessment and intervention program in high-risk patients—will result in better health outcomes.

The FORCE team sees the community based primary care provider as the leader in maintaining coordinated care for such patients, facilitated by an integrated care protocol that fosters continuity of care especially. A diagrammatic representation of this integrated, comprehensive approach to the management of patients with osteoporosis in Sault Ste. Marie is shown in Figure 11.3.

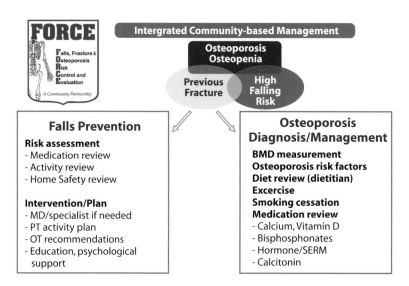

Figure 11.3: Schematic overview of a comprehensive care program for patients at risk from falling and fracturing with underlying osteoporosis. Adapted, with permission, from FORCE.

The principal outcomes measured in the FORCE project are assessments of the outcomes listed in Figure 11.3; that is, the appropriate management of falls and osteoporosis. Additional outcomes being measured across the community include a registry of falls and fractures, and patient activity levels, as well as patient satisfaction and quality of life analyses and assessments of patient education and treatment adherence.

I have visited Sault Ste. Marie in the context of this program and it was a most enlightening visit. As part of the agenda, I attended a meeting of FORCE's steering committee. It was an experience that reminded me very much of my previous experiences with the ICONS partners. The setting was a large conference room of the Sault Area Hospital. Many of the executives of the hospital were in attendance, along with the other partners. It was a remarkable blend of institutional and community based people committed to the study goals. The meeting was congenial, productive and efficient. Everyone seemed to know how best to contribute, when to speak and when to listen.

The meeting was chaired by Dr. Hui Lee, a general internist from the community. He was also the principal investigator and project officer for FORCE. He was a young man who had obvious respect and admiration from his peers and co-workers, which I think contributed significantly toward the visible commonality of the proceedings. I later served with Dr. Lee on a committee of the Ontario Ministry of Health and Long-term Care and got to know him better. He was bright, conscientious, collaborative and community-oriented. In 2002, for his work in the community, the College of Physicians and Surgeons of Ontario named him as the ideal physician.

I am greatly saddened by the fact that Dr. Hui Lee died suddenly in March 2004. His passing was a tragedy for his family and friends and his community. It is also a great loss for the advancement of the partnership and measurement model for improving health care in our country. There are few people with his vision and commitment. He was a champion who will be greatly missed. I hope his work and his example will not be lost to us.

Recognizing Osteoporosis and Its Consequences in Quebec (ROCQ)

Recognizing Osteoporosis and its Consequences in Quebec is the third large disease management project in osteoporosis that Merck Frosst has engaged in as a partner. Recently launched, the other partners in ROCQ include academic and community physicians from across Quebec and the industry (Aventis, Procter & Gamble, Lilly and Novartis).

Like the partnerships of MOMM and FORCE, the ROCQ team is driven by an appreciation for osteoporosis as a burden of illness in society and the large care gaps in diagnosing and treating this treatable disease, which carries such high risk for so many older women.

The project's approach to improving the diagnosis and treatment of osteoporosis in Quebec, like most other work in this field, is multiphased and projected to continue over several years. Briefly, sequential cohorts of patients with fragility fractures (a reliable clinical marker of osteoporosis) will be recruited and followed, and various interventions will be applied and evaluated to improve diagnostic and treatment patterns and patient outcomes (see Appendix K).

AIMS, MAAUI, CANOAR and CURATA

As exemplified in all the above projects, key features of modern disease management programs include a focus on the patient to optimize diagnosis, prescription, compliance and access; a shift from isolated inputs and individual agendas to multipartner systems views highlighting and benefiting from collaboration of all providers and patients; and creating and sharing new knowledge, particularly as it relates to the measurement and feedback of practices. This leads to improved health for whole populations.

Because it focuses on measuring and closing gaps between usual and best care and outcomes, the partnership/measurement model of disease management has the advantage of providing payers and users of health resources with a reassuring evidence base that we are or are not getting the best return for our health dollars. One area in which the Patient Health team at Merck Frosst has concentrated efforts in further defining appropriateness of care is in the use of anti-inflammatory medications, particularly their chronic use in disorders of the musculoskeletal system. Currently we are working with government, academic and community-based partners across the country on several innovative programs. These programs have provided us with some important insights that I would like to highlight here.

The Alberta Improvement for Musculoskeletal Disorders Study (AIMS) team's initial approach was to establish the burden of illness for such diseases in the province. They found that about 20 percent of all patient visits to caregivers involve seeking care for a musculoskeletal complaint. These patients are frequently in the working-age population (younger than sixty-five) and they are often male. They found that analysis of existing databases, as with chart audits, is complicated by the problem of missing or lack of specificity in recorded data. Notwithstanding, they found the single most frequent problem for which these patients seek care is chronic back pain.

Perhaps of most interest in the early AIMS analyses are the remarkable age-related differences in how and from whom patients seek care for their musculoskeletal problems (see Figure 11.4). Briefly, younger patients seem to favour consultations with chiropractors, while older patients seek care from physicians, particularly general and family practitioners. It seems the beliefs in the health belief model of care may change with age and experience.

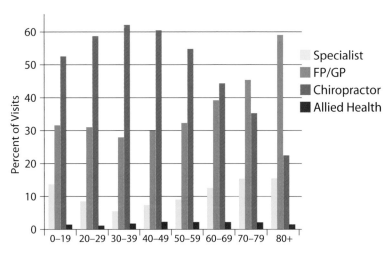

Figure 11.4: Distribution of care visits, by age of patient and type of provider, for patients with problems related to diseases of muscles, bones and joints in Alberta in 2001. The problems would range from back pain to muscle strains to the various types of arthritis. FP/GP refers to community-based physicians. Younger patients are predominantly treated by chiropractors. However, with increasing age, patients seek more care from medical doctors, either GPs or specialists, and decrease attendance at chiropractors' offices. Use of allied health personnel, such as physiotherapists, is relatively infrequent irrespective of age. Reproduced, with permission, from AIMS.

Ongoing initiatives of the AIMS project team include more detailed investigation of diagnoses in this field of musculoskeletal diseases and further assessments of treatment patterns, particularly as they relate to the evidence base around the optimum management of high- and low-risk patients.

The Manitoba Anti-inflammatory Appropriate Utilization Initiative (MAAUI) was designed with a first phase to determine prescribing patterns for chronic anti-inflammatory drug use across the province, irrespective of disease diagnosis and in anticipation of finding care gaps, with subsequent intervention phases to close the gaps. In the MAAUI study, patients who were older than sixty-five, or who had a previous history of peptic ulcer or bleeding disorder, or who required anticoagulants or blood thinners or steroid drugs or had other serious diseases were considered high-risk patients. Patients on chronic anti-inflammatory drugs in the absence of these risk factors were considered low-risk patients.

Based on the evidence for minimizing the risk of bleeding, ulcers or perforations in the stomach or intestines, guidelines for chronic anti-inflammatory drug use most often suggest that the best practice for high-risk patients is prescription of either a COXII inhibitor (COXIB) or a combination of a traditional non-steroidal anti-inflammatory drug (NSAIDs) with another drug designed to protect the gut from risky side effects. In MAAUI, prescription of either of these therapies in high-risk patients was considered appropriate therapy. In low-risk patients, prescription of the traditional NSAIDs was considered appropriate treatment. The findings of the database analysis of patients taking anti-inflammatory drugs between August 1, 1999 and September 30, 2000 are summarized in Figure 4.4.

Briefly, among the Manitoba patients taking chronic anti-inflammatory drugs, high-risk patients made up about more than 80 percent of all patients receiving chronic anti-inflammatory therapy and less than 20 percent were at low risk for bleeding and related complications in their stomach or intestines. In terms of therapeutic appropriateness, there were two care gaps. In high-risk patients, 53 percent were inappropriately treated with NSAIDs only. That is, they did not receive either COXIBs or protective combination therapy. Among low-risk patients, 44 percent were treated with COXIBs or combination therapy, which could be considered unnecessary overtreatment.

These findings from Manitoba are very similar to those from another large database analysis of a Nova Scotia seniors' population, using very similar definitions of patient risk and appropriateness of prescriptions. Taken together, they have certainly expanded my sense of how to better define appropriateness of care. In particular, some consideration of the level of patient risk may be necessary when considering whether one therapy versus another is appropriate or not.

In thinking about how to optimally and practically close care gaps, these studies suggest that intervention should include attacking both under-prescription of proven therapies in high-risk patients and over-prescription in low-risk patients. My sense, however, is we will make more progress in closing care gaps in high-risk patients because doctors will perceive a greater patient benefit and be more prepared to change patterns of undertreatment, compared to over-treatment of low-risk patients where the stimulus to prescribe may be over-safety, which they will not change easily despite the evidence. This theory remains to be proven in future studies, although the data from CURATA mentioned below tend to support this idea.

The Canadian Osteoarthritis Treatment Program (CANOAR) had a primary goal of determining the contemporary prescribing practices of a selected cohort of busy Ontario community care physicians. A secondary goal was to assess the potential influence of availability and type of reimbursement on prescription patterns. A very innovative feature of CANOAR was that measurements of all clinical data were directly entered in the doctors' offices at the time of patient visits.

CANOAR stressed the development of methods that busy physicians, with a high incidence of osteoarthritis patients in their practice, would find valuable in the routine care of these patients. Consequently, the community physicians' opinion and input into decisions about study design and implementation were highly valued. Diagnostic criteria, data forms, patient enrolment and communications processes were as simple as possible and guided by a pre-launch pilot test. This process enabled the substitution of the completed data form for the clinical chart note, if so desired. Anonymous data were faxed to the project data centre, where automated translation into electronic form, cleaning, encoding, aggregation, progress monitoring, monthly feedback reporting and analysis were performed. Over fourteen months, 119 Ontario doctors compiled data on 5,947 patients during 8,846 consecutive patient visits. In terms of anti-inflammatory drug-prescribing practices, 56 percent of these osteoarthritis patients were prescribed COXIBs and 44 percent received traditional drugs. Among patients with a history of a clinically significant stomach or intestinal complication, COXIB use was 66 percent, rising to 85 percent if the event was within the preceding two months.

Thirty-nine percent of the study patients had private insurance coverage for their medications. Interestingly, of the patients without private coverage, they were older, more likely to be women and to have more concomitant diseases and risk, including twice the number of risk factors for stomach and intestinal complications. Despite their greater risk, these patients were more likely to receive traditional NSAIDs only, compared to the lower-risk patients who had private-plan coverage. They were also less likely to receive COXIBs than patients with private-plan insurance.

These CANOAR data not only confirmed that care gaps are present in the management of osteoarthritis patients who receive anti-inflammatory drugs, they also suggested that, at least in part, the inappropriate prescription may be driven by the type of patient insurance coverage for drug reimbursement.

This becomes another issue to consider as we struggle to better define appropriateness of care and how to make it better.

As expressed frequently throughout this book, the desired endpoints in modern disease management are to close care gaps between the usual and the best care and gain improved patient outcomes. In such programs, the most commonly used interventions to improve provider prescribing practices and patient compliance are education, reminders, incentives and specifically measurement and feedback—the more the better. Evaluation of specific intervention tools, in specific disease settings, is still relatively uncommon. One of the most valuable innovations of the project called Concertation pour une Utilisation Raisonnée des Anti-Inflammatoires dans le Traitement de l' Arthtrose (CURATA), was to evaluate two educational interventions on the appropriate use of anti-inflammatory agents in patients with osteoarthritis (Beaulieu et al. 2004).

One intervention was an evidence-based treatment algo-rithm, printed on plasticized paper and distributed to physicians caring for patients with osteoarthritis (see Appendix L). The other intervention was an interactive workshop, conducted by specialists in bone and joint diseases and family physicians. It focused on realistic cases of osteoarthritis patients.

Two evaluations were made: a comparison of physicians' knowledge of the evidence-based treatment of osteoarthritis, as well as a comparison of physicians' prescribing patterns before and after the educational interventions. All study interven-tions were associated with improvement in practice patterns. The algorithm (see Appendix L) had the least beneficial effects, the workshop more and the combination the greatest. In terms of appropriateness, the interventions had a greater impact on improving the use of risk-reducing therapies for high-risk patients, and less impact on decreasing the overuse of these therapies in low-risk patients.

Thus, CURATA findings support previous work that indicates education is efficacious in improving prescribing practices, and that multiple interventions are better than single ones. Such an approach is preferable for any disease management project if it can be managed fiscally and physically.

The results of these contemporary applications of disease management processes in real-world practices—AIMS, MAAUI, CANOAR and CURATA—are complementary and consistent. There is a large burden of illness and fiscal demand created by patients taking anti-inflammatory drug therapy. High-risk patients outnumber low-risk patients by a ratio of about 4:1 and the dominant care gap is underuse of risk-reducing strategies. In low-risk patients, there is overuse of these same medications in a minority of patients. Educational interventions improve appropriateness of prescribing patterns, although further improvement is needed. Things can be better.

Diabetes Hamilton

Diabetes Hamilton is an initiative that Merck Frosst has only recently become aware of, but it began several years ago.

Diabetes is a metabolic disease thought of by most people to be a problem of high levels of sugar in blood. However, diabetes is more correctly characterized as a heart or blood vessel disease. That is because diabetic patients get sick and die from heart attacks, brain strokes, kidney failure and blindness as the blood vessels in these and other vital organs get clogged up with atherosclerosis, which restricts the blood supply. While diabetes is a disease of individuals, there are now so many people with diabetes—and the number is growing—that many health professionals consider diabetes a public health problem like a flu epidemic, AIDS or long-term SARS.

Certainly, the people who founded Diabetes Hamilton believe that diabetes is a public health issue. This partnership is led by Dr. Hertzel Gerstein, a medical specialist in diabetes treatment from Hamilton's McMaster University. The other partners include community-based family doctors and pharmacists, diabetes patient programs and organizations in the Hamilton area, optometrists, chiropodists, podiatrists, medical laboratories and specialty services, such as shoe stores that cater to diabetic patients with poor circulation in their feet.

Moreover, the Diabetes Hamilton team thinks that things can be better. The consequences of diabetes can be reduced. Their recommendations for reducing the risk from diabetes are summarized in Figure 11.5.

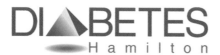

Reduce the consequences of diabetes	
A A1c:	good control of blood sugar
B BP:	good control of blood pressure
C Chol:	good control of blood fats like cholesterol
D Drugs:	ASA, ACE-I/ARB, statins, beta blockers, etc.
S Screen:	eyes, kidneys, feet
S Self-care:	patients' monitoring of therapy and lifestyle
S Self-efficacy:	patients' belief in self-management

Figure 11.5: The recommendations for reducing the cardiovascular complications that threaten the lives of diabetic patients. Adapted, with permission, from Diabetes Hamilton.

The problem in realizing the recommendations outlined in Figure 11.5 is that the standard form of primary medical care in most places is not designed for the ongoing care of a disease that may last for twenty or thirty years. In the traditional ideal clinical model of diabetes care, patients are referred most often by their family physician to a specialized health care team composed of physicians, nurses, dietitians, pharmacists, chiropodists, podiatrists, optometrists and social workers. The rising prevalence and burden of diabetes has, however, exposed a growing care gap between the need for such teams and their availability within many communities. Unfortunately, the vast majority of people with diabetes are not seen regularly in any specialized program and do not have systematic access to comprehensive and continuing diabetes expertise.

Diabetes Hamilton offers an alternative approach to care that broadens focus from provision of limited health care services in the traditional clinical setting to development of resources in the community at large. These resources are designed to be easily accessed by consumers who want to educate themselves and facilitate the self-management of their diabetes and its consequences.

Diabetes Hamilton focuses particularly on helping patients do whatever they can to reduce their own future risks and optimize their health, by providing patients with information and a sense of being empowered to seek or suggest that their care be optimized to reflect evidence-based comprehensive and seamless care. On a very practical level, Diabetes Hamilton has created a user-friendly inventory of community services for diabetic patients that guides access to resources to help patients follow their providers' recommendations and the recommendations outlined in Figure 11.5. This inventory, which contains clear and simple descriptions of services and joining instructions for more than 100 local resources, has now been distributed to 500 diabetes service providers, such as doctors, pharmacies and hospitals.

As of December 2003, Diabetes Hamilton had recruited 1,600 patients with diabetes and 300 local primary care physician members. It has sponsored displays at community fairs, pharmacies, service organizations and local supermarkets, as well as producing continuing education events and public education forums. And it has produced and distributed patient and provider newsletters on a quarterly basis (see Appendix M).

Diabetes Hamilton has, in addition, created a voluntary registry of people with diabetes, including an annual follow-up form to collect long-term information on diabetes risk factors and their change with interventions. The future plans of the team include developing on-line, electronic communication tools that allow participants to register and receive newsletters on-line, as well as further measurements of practices and patient outcomes.

This innovative community-oriented model was driven by the recognition that things could be better and there were existing resources available to make them better. The partnership has created a community-based Hawthorne Effect that is indeed making things better through the commitment of a broad array of stakeholders in the community, including individuals with diabetes expertise. These are people who are willing to assume local leadership by providing a simple means for linking and communicating all the community resources. It is an effective and compelling model. I believe it is transportable to other communities that are also dealing with this increasing public health issue.

I salute the Diabetes Hamilton team. They are making things better.

The other impression I took away from my initial briefing meeting with Dr. Gerstein was that, like me, he, too, has been on a professional journey. He had been traditionally trained in medical school, had specialty training and then entered an academic career in which he was very successful in his early research efforts. He discovered the value of participation in clinical trials for himself, his university and his patients. And then he seems to have realized that things could be even better for patients and was committed to make that happen.

In the future, the partnership-measurement model of patient health management will be secured by community leaders like Dr. Gerstein. I look forward to it. It can only make things better.

PART 3

WHAT HAVE WE LEARNED SO FAR?

Chapter 12

WHAT WORKS: THE ACTION PLAN

Recurring Themes

As I look back at the past and into the future, I am fairly certain that what worked in the past to improve care and outcomes will continue to work in the future.

There are some major recurring themes in successful patient health management as I see it. My top ten include the following:

1. Things can be better.
2. Care gaps are everywhere.
3. Commitment to intervene is a cornerstone of success.
4. Community-based partnerships are central to success.
5. Measurement and communication are key processes.
6. Hope is a powerful facilitator for better care and outcomes.
7. Improving care is an enabler—a call to arms for all stakeholders.
8. Anyone can do it.
9. Include rather than isolate.
10. Things will be better.

The Mantra: Things Can Be Better

The mantra that things can be better seems obvious in light of all the improvements in care and outcomes over the last ten years, particularly in our projects. I believe that things can always be better.

Just as obviously, many people believe that things can be better even before they see or experience the kind of evidence that the various projects have delivered. I mean people such as the nuns who first started focused patient health management in Canada and the many first-time participants, both patients and providers, in care improvement projects. Optimism that the future will be better is part of human nature.

However, pessimists do bring a point of view to things and it is important not to discount their opinions. I experienced a pertinent case of such pessimistic thinking about ten years ago. At that time, my colleagues and I were evaluating a clinical trial protocol designed to test whether a new therapy was efficacious for treating patients with acute heart attacks. The overwhelming majority opinion was that the trial was worthwhile to become involved with and to determine whether the new treatment was a better treatment. Somewhat disappointing for me was the dissenting opinion expressed by one of the younger physicians in our group. He thought there was no need for additional innovative therapy—that we already had enough proven therapies for these patients.

I do not know if this stated view was his primary reason for voting against the clinical trial, but what struck me at the time was his stated premise that what we have in terms of available therapy at any time in health care is good enough. And, by extension, good enough at any time is good enough for all time. This is not, however, thinking that will contribute to innovation and progress. From that viewpoint, it is dangerous thinking.

I wondered how many people in Caesar's time felt that their health care and average life expectancy were good enough. They must have been a minority or at least they did not represent the only opinion. If they had, then the greatly increased life expectancy that we enjoy today, much of which has occurred over the last half century, would have to be ascribed to some very favourable play of chance. Life expectancy just improved of its own accord.

Chance can certainly go in our favour half of the time, but we can continually facilitate and accelerate our health status by trying to innovate and improve.

There are still large care gaps in many of society's most burdensome illnesses. Things can always be better. It works as a very good starting point.

Commitment

I have often thought it is important to avoid feeling discouraged when seeing so many opportunities and thinking we have so few resources to take advantage of them all. Expressed another way, we should not let our inability to do everything stop or delay us from doing *something*. Don't drown in opportunity. Rather, commit to a single opportunity.

I think it is helpful to think of commitment in disease management as a twofold virtue; that is, there are really two levels of commitment in patient health management.

The first level is the commitment to make things better in terms of practices and outcomes. This is a crucial point in differentiating disease and patient health management as I understand it from outcomes research. It is the commitment to move beyond simply defining care gaps and their causes to taking action to fix the gaps.

The second level is to take action at a point or points in the health system that will likely result in significant and sustainable changes in practices and outcomes at the population level. On a practical basis, this means reaching out to community-based partners for help in finding and fixing care gaps. In fact, one could make the case that creating a community partnership is the first and main step in successful patient health management. It certainly has the additional benefits of conferring populist moral authority and accelerating the rate at which changes in population health will occur. If this approach is widely adopted for our most important and burdensome illnesses, I don't think we will have to wait twenty centuries to see improvements in care and outcomes equivalent to those that occurred between Caesar's time and ours.

There is another side to the commitment issue. To illustrate it best I will make an analogy to some recent public commitments from the national Canadian and American political scenes.

In 2004, Prime Minister Paul Martin declared war on waste and poor management in the federal government and stated his backing for an inquiry to find fault with the past and solutions for the future. U.S. President George W. Bush has recently declared space travel to the moon and Mars and an amendment to the Constitution regarding definition of marriage as national goals.

Whatever the merits of these various goals and proposals, I think there may well be backlash from the voter populations of each constituency if these stated goals are perceived as only talk without the will, energy and action—the commitment— to make them happen.

In patient health management, an equivalent risk would be to mount a project, create the partnership, define the care gap and then stop. A lesser risk would be stopping a successful project before sustainability was addressed and assured. Almost certainly, in each situation, there would be backlash from unmet expectations.

In health care, the commitment to make things better may have a long timeline and there may be a downside to not delivering when expectations have been raised.

Measurement and Communication

It is difficult to say enough about the value of communication and the particular value of communicating measured practices and outcomes. It is a powerful assistant in generating interest and stimulating the innovative thoughts and ideas to make things better. It sometimes takes courage for individuals to measure, compare and communicate their own or their group's practices and outcomes, but it usually can be managed in a collegial and anonymous, non-threatening manner.

If only one intervention could be applied in any particular disease management project, I would vote for measurements and their communication to providers. It works. Future care and outcomes will improve even if nothing else is done, at least for a time.

Communication is more than the feedback of practice data. It includes education of patients, providers and payers. It also embraces communication supports such as newsletters. It is anything that creates some of the sense of the value associated with membership in a community endeavour to improve health care. This sense of community membership is a very valuable asset in sustaining interest and persistent sense of value for involvement in a project that may run for several years.

Enabling Involvement—Patients Empowered

One of the most profound memories I carry with me from the ICONS experience is the sense of empowerment that developed among the patient participants in the project, particularly those who served on the steering committee. This seemed to me to be much more than an increased comfort level about speaking on medical matters because they had accrued a working knowledge of the medical issues of a specific disease, although that was probably part of it. It also involved some sense of responsibility to speak out on health policy matters in their town and their province. This compulsion to enter the health debate was driven by their sense of involvement. Beyond the clinical expertise gained, it extended to developing confidence that they could contribute significantly to the governance of a significant health initiative.

The Power of Hope

I think the belief that things *will* be better is an undervalued factor in health care management in the current environment. It is not new and is not often mentioned in glossaries of evidence-based care. But it seems to be a powerful virtue as it relates to patients' satisfaction with care and outcomes, particularly their quality of life.

Perhaps there is some way to blend and enhance the virtue with the evidence. This will require finding more evidence.

As I think through this issue and potential opportunity to make things better for patients, one continuing thought involves patient satisfaction surveys. The insights that I initially developed on the value of hope in improving patients' perception of quality of life came from such surveys. My sense is that we are not doing enough patient satisfaction surveys of our daily or usual practices. We are probably missing valuable insights from patients, particularly as patients are increasingly educated in diseases and their treatment. I have come to think of such surveys as a regular opportunity to improve concordance between providers and patients about many issues in health care, sort of an extension of the value of concordance in improving patient compliance with prescriptions. Perhaps this is feasible if facile survey tools can be developed. It is something worth pursuing.

Combining versus Isolating

There are many different simple ways to categorize people and processes in any area of endeavour. For example, one of my colleagues often speaks of two kinds of people at meetings: cooperators and competitors.

In health care, I have often thought that players, be they payers, providers or patients, were either isolators or combiners or, in simpler jargon, splitters versus lumpers. Briefly, splitters tend to break up concepts and problems into many smaller parts and keep them there. Lumpers tend to group issues and problems and seek partnership and integrated solutions, taking pride and comfort in an integrated approach and the contributions of others.

For example, in the area of compliance or patient adherence to medications, splitters might regard this issue exclusively as patients' responsibility and expect them to sort out any solutions. Lumpers more likely would consider the issues to be the responsibility of a number of players and plans to fix things would have better success if all the potential players—including patients, doctors, pharmacists, nurses, dietitians—were involved in defining and solving the problems. Another example is in the design and governance of a patient health project. Splitters might be inclined to keep all decision making within a small expert group and attempt to sell a baked cake to all the other parties needed to mount a successful project—the patients, community health professionals and government people. Lumpers, on the other hand, involve everybody from the beginning and work to make sure that everyone had a defined contribution from the start.

I think the idea of lumpers and splitters is also relevant to usual clinical care. Traditional solo practice is closer to the splitting concept; group practice or multisectoral practice is closer to the lumping concept. My prediction is that as we acquire more knowledge and skills, the effective lumping of our expertise will be increasingly valued. That is, the health care providers who are best able to regroup our health providers so they deliver the best and tailored comprehensive care in a continuous and flexible manner will be the most appreciated and successful—at least as judged by patients. So, as we go forward, I think lumping and sharing our talents and opportunities will go a long way toward making things better.

Chapter 13

WHAT DOESN'T WORK

Perhaps, for context, it would be wise to review the four basic things that have been repeatedly shown to improve practices and outcomes in disease management programs. They are measurement and feedback, education, reminders and incentives.

As indicated in the previous chapter, measurement, feedback, reminders and education might all be lumped under communication. If so, then productive disease management interventions might well be boiled down to communication and incentives.

In this context, incentives usually refer to financial incentives, for example, paying health care providers or patient consumers when they adhere better to best-practice guidelines in prescribing and complying with proven therapies. It works. It is used by some government public payers to improve adherence with guidelines: for example, in improving immunization practices and fostering the comprehensive management of diabetes. But like all interventions, it is not a silver bullet; it does not completely fix every care gap.

There seems to be something of a double or variable standard regarding the concept of financial incentives in health care and its management. For example, there are differing opinions as to whether it is acceptable or desirable for some people to make profits by selling prescription drugs across international borders. The same people may have different views on financial incentives, depending on whether the incentive is being provided by a public or private payer. Overall, it is fair to say there is no consensus at this time on the use of financial incentives in improving health care in Canada.

So, at least for the time being, until the public debate on financing enters the defining stage, we will be better served by avoiding any new and direct financial incentives to improve practices in disease management programs.

It is not that they won't work. They do work, but they may carry too much baggage at the present time and tend to distract people from the non-financial incentives that are available, such as measurement, education, sense of empowerment and achievement.

Is There Anything to Be Avoided?

No single process or intervention in disease management jumps to my mind as something to be avoided at all costs. In fact, the only real risk is to *not* do anything in patient health management. And to keep things in a positive framework, perhaps a better way to structure this section would be to summarize some practical imperatives for patient health management:

- Do something.
- Create manageable teams.
- Set realistic objectives.
- Expect incremental, not revolutionary, improvements.
- Be flexible.
- Favour practical rather than theoretical approaches and solutions.
- Think locally in buy-in and impact.
- Share experiences, results and governance.

However, some balance may be needed for optimal program performance. For example, it may be necessary to balance the sense of community authority, buy-in and empowerment that comes from a large steering committee with the need to get things done. A seventy-member self-directed work team may just drift. Somebody has to lead and oversee administration, so for efficiency, there should be an executive champion group.

It is also probably prudent to avoid setting unreasonable goals for untrained members, particularly for timelines and particularly early in a project's cycle. Rather, it is preferable to recognize the need for training and experience, both of which take time, to help make things better in the long term.

It is also wise to avoid the expectation that the particular project, no matter how good, will be a breakthrough, that it will answer all the problems of care and outcomes for any specific disease state in any specific place. Rather, it is much more likely that incremental innovations and progress will be made and future partnerships and projects will be necessary for future advances.

I would also advise avoiding too much rigidity in key processes, for example, how measurements are collected or how education and communications are delivered. I remember debating how the data management in ICONS and other projects would be conducted. Some players favoured an entirely electronic process for measurements and their transmission; others favoured a hard copy approach. However, what seems to be the best approach is a flexible process that best serves the individuals making and communicating the measurements. If they want paper records or electronic records, or both, a flexible system that serves their needs provides the greatest member satisfaction.

In fact, too much mandated uniformity should be avoided in general. That is, every intervention need not be applicable for every local setting. This is a somewhat heretical concept because in total quality management, from which we have borrowed many of our ideas, variation is usually thought of as a bad thing. In patient health management, however, at the community level, some small area variation might be a good thing. What works in Chicoutimi may not work in Lethbridge. But having the measurements of outcomes, before and after intervention, for each setting provides assurance that any differences or similarities will be detected, evaluated and compared. Certainly allowing for regional variation and flexibility is one practical way to broaden stakeholder buy-in.

Lastly, I think the partnership members should avoid any tendency to think that their experiences, achievements or failures are not valuable for others to know about. It is useful to publish or otherwise propagate results as widely and expeditiously as possible so that best practices can be adopted with less delay than in the past. In other words, there are at least two components or levels of being a true centre of excellence in disease management. The first level is attained by committing to build the partnership and implement the processes that make things better and creating a core of expertise and knowledge that leads to demonstrably better practices and outcomes. The second level is achieved when the created knowledge is disseminated so that others can use it to improve practices and outcomes.

An analogy might be that one half of a centre of excellence is like a castle of best practices without a working drawbridge. True excellence comes only when the castle's expertise crosses the drawbridge to the whole community outside the knowledge centre, particularly if it is accompanied by the commitment to intervene to make things better.

In summary, what is to be avoided is too much control or containing tendencies in the governance of patient health management programs and the propagation of their knowledge of how to make things better. These programs will be judged more successful when they are viewed as populist, activist endeavours rather than simply knowledge-generating exercises.

PART 4

VISION FOR THE FUTURE

Chapter 14

THE STRATEGIC ALTERNATIVES

One alternative is always not to do anything different, to maintain the status quo. However, in the current health care debate, that seems not to be a favoured or acceptable option. The perception is that too much is broken in terms of quality, access and costs in our health system to credibly argue for doing nothing.

What Could Feasibly Be Done Differently to Make Things Better?

Everybody would like to see better quality of care, including improved patient access to and use of products and services, and better outcomes at reduced total costs to the payers, the citizens of Canada.

Realistically, it is difficult for me to think of closing care gaps in diagnosis and therapy, as well as financing newer innovations from research and training new generations of providers, at lower cost than we incur now. We will have to spend more for health care as time passes.

Jeffrey Simpson of the *Globe and Mail* noted in a recent editorial entitled "Who Will Start a Frank Debate on Health Care?" that the additional money needed for health care can come only from Canadians' pockets, either through higher taxes or by allowing individuals to buy more health services from private sources. Administrative reforms and the wider institution of best practices—although good in themselves and being accomplished now—will not solve the issue of our health care system's sustainability.

A third possibility for increased money for health care would involve some combination of increased taxes and increased private sourcing of services.

As Simpson points out, the funding debate in meaningful terms has yet to be started, so I would like to put aside how we will fund the increased costs and move to how we might be assured of best return on value for whatever funds are available.

This desire for assurance and accountability for money spent brings us back to measurement. We need to measure what we are buying in terms of outcomes, as Nova Scotia Minister of Health Boudreau said many years ago at the launch of ICONS. And, we need to comfortably relate the gains in health outcomes for many people with chronic illnesses, through improved access, prescription and compliance practices, to gains in our productivity and competitiveness as a nation.

The simplest solution is to do more patient health management projects in more diseases and more places.

This would be useful, but I think it may not of itself be a bold enough or broad enough or deep enough strategy to ensure continuous quality improvement and sustainability of our health system. Although the concepts of partnership and measurement are simple, their creation, maintenance and advancement are not. It takes courage, commitment and perseverance. It requires skills in leadership and communication to deal with complex issues and environments. So, at least at this time, not everyone will sign up for patient health management. Nonetheless, for those who wish to begin or advance down this path, I hope this book will serve as a stimulus and a guide.

For others who might and could contribute to making things better in health care, we must enhance their chances of recognizing the effectiveness, cost efficiency and feasibility of patient health management. And we must also facilitate the development and availability of the necessary skills so that this potential pool of players can become bigger and better.

Beyond Patient Health Management

During the latter part of my tenure at the University of Alberta, Dr. Garner King delegated me to represent the Faculty of Medicine on a committee that was looking at the feasibility of consolidating management programs throughout the university. At the time, management programs were operating in several faculties, including business, education, engineering, health sciences and medicine, and the committee membership represented all of these areas.

As part of the exercise, we interviewed previous graduates of the various management programs, particularly people who had taken master's-level training in programs such as business administration or public administration. This group of interviewees included some very accomplished people who were then in very senior management positions, for example, deputy ministers of provincial government departments.

I found this part of the process very interesting and enlightening. The former graduates were engaging and interested in our goals. They had impressive personalities and accomplishments. They willingly offered their views based on their experience. They recognized and gave great credit to their formal management training as a valuable part of their career success. It seemed obvious to me that each person in his or her specific area had had very similar exposure to or training in the general principles and practices of management.

What I found jarring was that none of these very well-trained and successful people, who had trained in the same university in the same time frame, knew or communicated regularly with any of their counterparts. Moreover, and I guess not unexpectedly given the above, they had little appreciation for the goals, aspirations and issues of each other's professions, despite sharing similar grounding in management theory and practice. I began to think of this situation as something of a lost opportunity.

For example, it struck me that if the deputy minister of health and the deputy minister of finance in any province knowingly shared a common management experience and evidence base, they might work together more effectively to attain common and mutually supportive goals such as simultaneously improving the health and wealth of the province. At least their shared values would tend to foster a system approach, as opposed to a silo or component approach, to issues and solutions.

As a practical suggestion, I wondered whether the university should consider a common first year of management training during which all students, regardless of their final specialization, would experience the same classes and teachers in the same environment. In the second and successive years, the students would move to their specific areas of expertise in education, business, medicine, and so on. My sense was that, even after the immersion into their specialty, the students and future managers would carry with them an understanding and respect for their colleagues in the diversity of management areas. Part of that positive carry-over would include the comfort that comes from dealing with someone with shared experiences.

The idea gained no traction, as they say. Perhaps the time has come to resurrect some of these concepts of common management training and experience in the context of making things better in health care. "Everything has its time," as Dr. Garner King used to say.

Out of the Wilderness

I am not the only one thinking along these lines. A few years ago, I met Dr. Brenda Zimmerman, who at that time was an associate professor at McGill's School of Management in Montreal. Dr. Zimmerman's particular areas of interest and

expertise were in leadership and strategy, and she was especially focused on the health care arena. She is currently on the
faculty of the Schulich School of Business at York University in
Toronto, where she is leading the development of the Health
Industry Management Program.

Dr. Zimmerman and her Schulich colleagues recognize
that the health industry is a complex conglomeration of entities. It involves traditional entities such as hospitals and
long-term care institutions and players such as doctors, nurses, pharmacists, public health agencies, patients and patient
advocacy groups. But it also embraces other groups and institutions, including governments, the innovative research
community of pharmaceutical, medical device and biotech
companies, the media, venture capitalists, the legal and
insurance professions, charities and organized labour.

The overarching roles that are envisioned for this broad
array of health industry stakeholders include, in the Schulich
view, those of providers, suppliers, intermediaries, funders,
"framers", advocates, researchers and, ultimately, the principal
beneficiaries, the patients (see Figure 14.1).

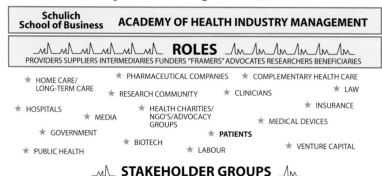

Figure 14.1: Graphic representation of the multiple stakeholders in the health
care arena or industry and the spectrum of roles they may play in an overlapping
or competing fashion at any time. Reproduced, with permission, from Dr. Brenda
Zimmerman, Health Industry Management Program, Schulich School of Business,
York University.

In Dr. Zimmerman's view, part of the complexity in health care
is due to the competing goals of some of the players. This line of

reasoning extends to suggest that part of the complexity is also the result of the missed opportunities inherent in the overarching but unseen and unknown similar management challenges of the various stakeholders. The overriding driving force of the new Schulich health management hypothesis is that more tools and enabling skills than are learned in traditional clinical environments are needed to reach the full potential of the medical and scientific innovations of our times.

In particular, Dr. Zimmerman and her colleagues believe that cross-disciplinary, cross-clinical and cross-sectoral discussions will deepen our understanding of the health industry.

These discussions will expose the multiple perspectives of the varied stakeholders, including the various biases and working assumptions of each component stakeholder group. The increased self-awareness, combined with the increased awareness of other stakeholders' roles, values and skills generated by the crossover experience, will lead to better understanding of health care issues and better solutions, even for problems that are now considered difficult or intractable. They believe that things can be better.

To practically achieve their goals, the team at Schulich has developed two initial courses: *International Healthcare Systems* and *Understanding the Canadian Health Industry: the Roles, Responsibilities and Challenges to Improve Health*. Both are positioned primarily for master's-level students in management. Currently, these courses have students enrolled from several clinical disciplines, including medicine and nursing. In the latter course, representatives from across the health industry are invited to share their experience with the students, to review the students' analyses and to be interviewed by the students to expose the underlying driving values, metaphors and decision making criteria of the different stakeholder groups.

The school's long-term goals include extended practical and theoretic collaboration with Canadian and American clinical schools and continued course development, leading to a broad-based two-year program culminating in an MBA degree in health management. Currently, a pilot program is being developed in association with Dartmouth Medical School in New Hampshire. This is an example of bridging the gaps in connection within the industry. Nurses, hospital managers and MBA students work together in a ten-week program to improve the effectiveness of selected clinical microsystems, including current measurement, feedback and feed-forward information systems. In complexity terms, the Schulich-Dartmouth partnership is attempting to create relationships in which the outcomes are driven less by what was initially brought to the table and more by the relationships and connections generated by the partnership. With truly generative relationships, it is difficult to reliably predict *a priori* what outcomes are achievable or even how to create them. It is a process that emerges from the creativity and mutual respect of cooperating partner members working toward an important goal.

One possibile way for candidates in such a program to attain the preferred practical experience is to act as project officers or managers in a patient health management program such as the Improving Cardiovascular Outcomes in Nova Scotia or the Manitoba Anti-inflammatory Appropriate Use Initiative. The optimal performance of people in this role requires daily interaction with many different sections of the health system, including all of the clinical and academic players, as well as many of the administrative and political players and payers. To be successful, the project managers must understand the value of the many skills necessary to make up a successful team: vision, facilitation, monitoring and closing/finishing. They must be also be able to lead, to take people where they might not otherwise go and to close care gaps at the community level. The opportunity to see, experience, learn and teach many facets of the health system is real and gratifying in such a role, but it is also challenging.

Another innovative cross-sectoral program in health care is McGill's MD/MBA program. It is a joint project of the schools of medicine and management. The program trains students entering medical school in both business and medicine over the course of several years, culminating in a joint degree, the MD/MBA.

I have had some exposure to the program and its students over the course of the last few years through symposia and summer practical experiences. The students are extremely intelligent and keen to have a broader than usual education. For example, Christopher Wahl, currently entering the third year of this program, combined his medical and business interests and skills during a summer session with us in the Patient Health Department to help develop our review of, and future strategy for, closing gaps in patient compliance or treatment adherence (Wahl et al. 2004).

The combined business and medical program at McGill is, however, the only one presently operational in Canada and is limited to only six students per year. I have heard that a similar program will also shortly be developed at the University of Western Ontario and the Ivey School of Business. However, even if Ivey comes on board and rapidly adopts and attains the goals and benchmarks of the Schulich and McGill programs in advancing cross-sectoral awareness, respect and formal training and skills acquisition in many aspects of our health system, they are unlikely by themselves to produce a national or sustained institutional effect. Things can surely be better, but more is needed.

The findings of the Clinical Quality Improvement Network investigators with regard to doctors' intentions to practice based on evidence are worth reviewing in the present context. Briefly, when many factors were considered, the CQIN findings suggested that the one factor most highly associated with best treatment intentions was the time that had elapsed since doctors had completed their undergraduate or their MD training. The more recently they had completed this training, the more closely their practice patterns reflected best practices as defined by the evidence of randomized clinical trials, so training or education was obviously important in promoting best practices.

And the training that doctors received in their undergraduate medical school years seemed particularly powerful or influential in their practice decisions.

Yet very little of what is covered in this book is covered in the curricula of contemporary medical school training. The degree to which the concepts of the care gap and, to my knowledge, the methods of closing it are taught in pharmacy or nursing schools is also limited. I am not aware of any institution or groups of institutions that are offering common teaching of the core values of teams, including cross-sectoral membership and leadership, in improving provider practices and patient outcomes.

So, there is an opportunity to make things better in undergraduate education, with the goal of putting patients first. At a practical level, I think that consideration should be given to formalizing crossover training of some of the major clinical disciplines such as medicine, nursing and pharmacy. During the communal training, I think that students should be exposed to the concepts of system management, leadership and strategy skills and the value of working in teams, as well as more specific training in public and population health, particularly the omnipresent care gaps, and, of course, the partnership-measurement model of disease management as one promising solution to make things better.

To get a further perspective on the issues and opportunities of changing our concepts of and methods in training the health care professionals of the future, I have asked Dr. Brenda Zimmerman to provide her assessment of what may be possible. She writes:

> I share Dr. Montague's optimism about what is possible in health care. The Schulich program is a way of demonstrating our optimism. I have had people say to me that the reason multi-sector approaches to health education don't exist is because they won't work. That remains to be seen.

In my view, what we are trying to do is both essential and achievable. If we are at the cusp of a truly patient-centred concept of health care, it is essential for participants in the health industry to more deeply understand and respect the value each brings to health and health care. Patient-centred care requires truly effective coordination across functions and sectors. This is challenging, but not impossible to achieve. We have skills, research and approaches to teach stakeholder mapping and self-awareness. We have sophisticated literature on team effectiveness and building coherence while expanding diversity. There is an increased understanding that revealing one's assumptions, biases and implicit or explicit metaphors is a key management skill when dealing with diverse populations and complex contexts. We know about the power of paradox in complex systems and are not shocked by the idea that self-interest and collective interest can co-exist or that sustainable systems need both cooperation and competition.

To close the care gap, we need to recognize that creativity and accountability can co-exist.

Great progress has been made and will be made by not only studying the problems but also examining what is working and probing why. There are methods—for example, appreciative inquiry—to teach this mode of thinking as a complement to our traditional problem-solving approaches. We don't know the answers, but we know how to pose the questions in ways that will reveal better answers. These are teachable skills. Hence I am optimistic that we can educate ourselves, those new to the health industry and those who have been in it for some time in the techniques needed to address the care gap. It won't be easy. But everything has its time and the timing is now right for movement across traditional health sector boundaries in understanding and education. Things can be better.

Chapter 15

SKATE TO WHERE THE PUCK WILL BE: WAYNE GRETZKY'S STRATEGIC PLAN

"I skate to where I think the puck will be," is what Wayne Gretzky is reported to have replied when asked how he played hockey the way he did, and what his plan was. Mr. Gretzky's reply is perhaps the most succinct and clear strategic plan ever enunciated. It was also extremely successful.

At first glance, it would appear that the trick to successfully implementing this simple plan was Mr. Gretzky's unparalleled gift of being able to reliably predict where the puck would be much of the time.

If we adapt this analogy to the debate on the future of Canadian health care, the immediate question becomes: Do we have a Gretzky-level degree of certainty about where the puck will be? Obviously, uncertainty arises. With uncertainty comes a tendency to do nothing just because we are not certain of success. Of course, not even Wayne Gretzky was right all the time. Sometimes he did not know where the puck was going to be. Nonetheless, it did not stop him from pursuing his plan.

Recently there has been much reported in the media concerning the political and economic relations between Canada and the United States. One theme that has repeatedly arisen in this plethora of current public opinion from both sides of the border is that Canadians are often seen as "ditherers." That is, we have a hard time deciding and following up with action on important issues such as national and continental security and our military's state and role.

I cannot help but think that with regard to health care and its sustainability, we are also dithering. We have seen several provincial and national commissions formally investigate and report on health system issues and preferred solutions over the last several years. However, there has been no meaningful or focused action across the nation. The debates are still continuing and continue to be focused more on process, particularly the processes of governance and funding, than on care and outcomes. It sometimes strikes me that the Medicare sustainability process is replacing the Navy's helicopter sustainability process as the poster child for Canadian public sector decision making.

With a second look, I think it is important to realize that an important compelling message in the Gretzky strategy statement is the concept of action ("I skate"), while thinking of the way the future will likely unfold. In fact, for me, this commitment to action may be the most relevant and easily transferable idea from Mr. Gretzky's hockey strategy to a strategy for sustaining health care. So how can willing and able individuals sustain and improve health care and outcomes while we are thinking and debating? Some suggestions are:

- Finance ministers learn the value to the economy of improved health outcomes and see the money spent on improving care and outcomes as investments in a better economic future for Canada.
- Health ministers support team- and community-based partnerships in health knowledge creation and dissemination and use the information gained to promote evidence-based policies and resource allocations.
- Health and finance ministers commit, like Minister Boudreau at the launch of ICONS, to manage by outcomes, not by costs alone.

- Physicians and other providers explore the value of team approaches in education and implementation of health care.
- Patients accept, value and make more contributions toward governance decisions and their accountability in health care.

Certainly, one thing that can be done using current resources and keeping within all existing principles of Medicare and political tensions, is for like-minded people to form a partnership and measure practices and outcomes around a disease burden that is important for them and their community. They can build their own ICONS. It is not rocket science. It is doable. It is hard, but it is rewarding. Most tools are available or importable. Commitment must, however, come from the local trenches.

I am confident that as the health care future unfolds, disease management philosophy, with its focused application of resources, will increasingly be an integral part of the strategy and practice of health care. It fills a need. In fact, as my colleague John Sproule says, you could make a case that the ultimate underlying need that patient health management satisfies is that it successfully broadens our health system from a dominant focus on acute care to a focus that addresses the enlarging need to deal with chronic illnesses.

One critical part of a system that shifts from a "treat to street" acute-care focus to a focus that successfully manages chronic care is the adoption of continuous measurement and communication of important system parameters. The partnership measurement model of patient health management is particularly well-suited to address this requirement for success. A comforting upside of such measurements in the context of uncertainty is that they will reduce uncertainty and increase accountability for future decisions.

My sense is that we will continue to find innovative ways to group resources so that we can effectively and efficiently meet patient-customer needs for more comprehensive and continuous care. I predict that the next big advances in disease management in Canada will be along the lines of groups of disease management or comprehensive care management. And the most successful of these will be the ones that best match the groups of diseases that real-world patients suffer from.

For example, a comprehensive care program that simultaneously manages heart disease and depression seems like a good bet because of the high overlap of these two diseases in the same patients. Or, similarly, a program that focused on diabetes, obesity and heart disease might be attractive to many patients since it would not only be realistically comprehensive but also allow for continuity of care, starting even before any symptoms of any disease state developed and continuing for as long as the patient or his/her family wanted.

Other possible examples of innovative disease management programs along these lines might be a women's health initiative, in which diseases like osteoporosis, arthritis and heart disease might be grouped with optimal nutritional and social and economic advice and support. Perhaps most attractive of all would be an elderly health initiative, with a simple goal of making care and practices for older patients as evidence-based and population effective as care for younger patients.

Do Something

When I am asked why I wrote this book, I have an answer.

I began this book as a reflective journey through my working life because I thought I had learned some things that might be helpful or at least interesting to others. And I felt compelled to tell them.

However, as I was in the process of writing, a colleague who read the draft manuscript asked me some questions for which I had no ready answers. They were not about why I wrote the book. They were about why I did what I did that led to the writing of the book. Specifically, he asked why I had moved away from the more usual clinical or academic medical careers, which focus on individual patient outcomes and the traditional university-based pursuit of excellence, to choose a path that might best be described as interventional epidemiology, committed to improving the outcomes of whole populations. He went on to ask if there was a single event that drove me in that direction.

I have repeatedly searched for the answers to these questions, and not only to improve my own insight. I think it is also important for readers to understand as well as possible where I am coming from as I offer recommendations and solicit support for a future health care strategy. Off the top, I would say the answer is not simple or single. It lies in some combination of recognizing the challenge and opportunity presented by care gaps, thinking that things can be better and realizing that I might never have any equal or second chances to make them better.

When I look back, I realize I am fortunate to have had three distinct and rewarding careers. I was first an army officer, then an academic physician and most recently an executive in the health industry. I have enjoyed each career and learned much in each. I am proud of all these professions and career experiences. Perhaps above all else, I am proud of and thankful for the people I have met in these various life stages and careers. It has been a great privilege, and I have been very lucky.

One of the people who impressed me most in my professional journey was a young cardiologist named Norman Davies whom I met when I moved to Edmonton in 1988. Norman was perhaps the most gifted person I have ever encountered, anywhere. He was intellectually brilliant, nearly without peers. Consistently, he was the class leader in all his formal education, from grade school to medical school. He was also greatly gifted musically. He had been a professional jazz and symphonic percussionist prior to entering medical school and he continued to play for pleasure all his life.

217

However, it was humanness that set Norman truly apart. He was funny and graceful. He loved conversation, both talking and listening. He took joy in the accomplishments and experiences of others. He had a sense of integrity to match his intellectual skills. He demonstrated great love for his family. He was compassionate and caring about his patients. And he was absolutely passionate about Wayne Gretzky and the Oilers. He could, and did, recollect hundreds of individual plays of Gretzky and his teammates in specific games over many years.

Yet, more than once I walked around with him in the outdoor hospital parking lot in the early evening cold of an Edmonton winter, frantically searching for his car so we could go home. This great man, who had a photographic memory for many things, routinely forgot exactly where he had parked his car twelve hours earlier.

It took me a while to think through these apparent contradictions in Norman's character. In fact, there were no contradictions. Norman remembered only what was important. And, as he said to me one day in the spring of 1991: "From now on, I am only going to work on things that are important." He was focusing and he was committing. At that time, he was specifically referring to seeing the SCAT trial through to completion and enhancing our group's participation in the national cardiology residency training program. I was impressed by his statement and I thought it was very unusual for someone so young. Norman was thirty-seven at the time.

He died suddenly two months later while jogging one night and, unfortunately, never had the opportunity to pursue his strategic plan over the long term and see the rewards. The nation, particularly the health care sector, lost a great talent with the premature death of Norman Davies. Often it is hard to find the silver lining in such an obvious dark cloud.

But I never forgot Norman's commitment to focus on important things. And I always remember it in the context of our human frailty, particularly our inability to reliably predict the future.

Norman died before we established our strategic direction in disease management to close care gaps. However, I am pretty certain he would have thought it was important work—important enough to work at. And when I think about the issues surrounding the care gap, I am also reminded of Norman when I consider our opportunity to close care gaps. I am particularly stimulated by thinking we should take advantage of our opportunities and act when we can—now.

We have no guarantee that we will have the luxury to wait for a better time. And neither do a lot of the patients we could help by doing something—now—to make things better.

Appendices

APPENDIX A

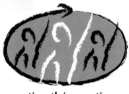

gestion thérapeutique
patient health

Guiding Principles for Public/Private Partnerships: Disease Management and Outcomes Research

As strong proponents of industry/government/academia/community partnerships in population health that are in the public and corporate interests, Merck Frosst Canada Ltd. wishes to articulate the principles of institutional ethics and institutional dissemination by which it navigates.

Partnerships Fostering Open Communication, Transparency and Trust

- Vision: The Best Health for the Most People at the Best Cost.
- Partnership-based outcomes research and disease management allow Canada's Rx&D companies to participate fully with other stakeholders in the health care system—universities, hospitals, physicians, pharmacists, employers, employees, the insurance industry, patients and governments across Canada—to ensure patient access to optimal therapies, while improving costs and health outcomes.
- From an institutional ethics viewpoint, the guiding principles are: an enduring value system of broad stakeholder

partnerships, outcomes measurements and advocacy of evidence-based therapy. In this value system, equal valuing of all partners' contributions is paramount to success.

• In particular, multi-directional transparency of project processes and governance, including funding, data acquisition, data handling and data dissemination in all of its research collaborations, is strongly advocated.

• In all project partnerships, formal rules around data analysis and publication are fostered. The working principles are: the data belongs to the project/study, and, data management is overseen by the formal governance structures of the project/study, usually a multiple-person data management committee that determines the exact processes for acquiring, interrogating and propagating the data and its interpretations.

• No veto, or delay, of publication of data results by academic partners is sought. Rather, the most rapid dissemination of results that is scientifically feasible is encouraged.

Protocols

• Goal: Most disease management projects seek to close the gap between best care and usual care, so population outcomes (effectiveness) better reflect clinical trials results (efficacy), using the best available protocol.

• All partners provide input to specific research questions, design and analysis. The project council, or steering committee, a multiple stakeholder group of the principal academic, industry, governmental and community partners, is the principal governance structure. It has decision power over protocol issues, within the framework of any pre-existing contracts or project charters.

• Pharmaceutical companies have a fiduciary responsibility to protect their property and image. As responsible corporate citizens, companies will not enter into research partnerships that are likely to yield inaccurate data acquisition, management or interpretation that are not in either public or private interests.

Data Dissemination

- Companies have a commitment to the measurement and feedback of health outcomes, costs, and processes. These are continually measured and communicated to providers to promote more efficacious care and use of resources. Thus, internal publication of data is an important first intervention tool to drive future improved practice patterns and patient outcomes.
- As indicated above, companies support the right of researchers to unencumbered external communication of full and complete results arising from partnership projects to advance scientific knowledge and direct policy development. Companies encourage these publications, with the usual request that the researchers provide copies of publications or presentations thirty (30) days prior to publication or presentation. Data always remains property of the study/project, not the companies.

Public Interest

- There is increasing evidence that consistent, long-term evidence-based approaches to disease management can significantly improve practice patterns and patient outcomes, including increased utilization of proven therapies and enhanced duration and quality of life, as well as incurring system savings or cost avoidance.
- A reasonable expectation is that governments will sustain successful projects in the long term. These decisions will be taken if the methods and processes, including the broad partnership and internal dissemination of data, drive improved patient outcomes and cost efficiencies that are in the public interest.
- The public interest is well served scientifically by the large body of data that is published, in an unencumbered and timely fashion, around each disease state project.
- Our company remains committed to public/private partnerships and process principles, as outlined above. It is part of our overall commitment to the scientific advance and the public interest of this nation.

223

APPENDIX B
Patient Management Template, Heart Function Clinic, circa 1994

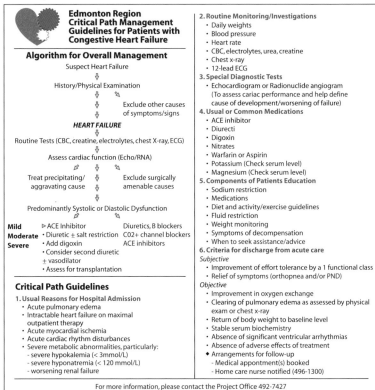

Edmonton Region Critical Path Management Guidelines for Patients with Congestive Heart Failure

Algorithm for Overall Management

Suspect Heart Failure
⇩
History/Physical Examination
⇩
⇩ ↘ Exclude other causes
⇩ of symptoms/signs
HEART FAILURE
⇩
Routine Tests (CBC, creatine, electrolytes, chest X-ray, ECG)
⇩
Assess cardiac function (Echo/RNA)
↙ ⇩ ↘
Treat precipitating/ ⇩ Exclude surgically
aggravating cause ⇩ amenable causes
⇩
Predominantly Systolic or Diastolic Dysfunction
↙ ↘

Mild	▷ ACE Inhibitor	Diuretics, B blockers
Moderate	• Diuretic ± salt restriction	CO2+ channel blockers
Severe	• Add digoxin	ACE inhibitors
	• Consider second diuretic ± vasodilator	
	• Assess for transplantation	

Critical Path Guidelines

1. Usual Reasons for Hospital Admission
- Acute pulmonary edema
- Intractable heart failure on maximal outpatient therapy
- Acute myocardial ischemia
- Acute cardiac rhythm disturbances
- Severe metabolic abnormalities, particularly:
  - severe hypokalemia (< 3mmol/L)
  - severe hyponatremia (< 120 mmol/L)
  - worsening renal failure

2. Routine Monitoring/Investigations
- Daily weights
- Blood pressure
- Heart rate
- CBC, electrolytes, urea, creatine
- Chest x-ray
- 12-lead ECG

3. Special Diagnostic Tests
- Echocardiogram or Radionuclide angiogram
  (To assess cariac performance and help define cause of development/worsening of failure)

4. Usual or Common Medications
- ACE inhibitor
- Diurecti
- Digoxin
- Nitrates
- Warfarin or Aspirin
- Potassium (Check serum level)
- Magnesium (Check serum level)

5. Components of Patients Education
- Sodium restriction
- Medications
- Diet and activity/exercise guidelines
- Fluid restriction
- Weight monitoring
- Symptoms of decompensation
- When to seek assistance/advice

6. Criteria for discharge from acute care
Subjective
- Improvement of effort tolerance by a 1 functional class
- Relief of symptoms (orthopnea and/or PND)

Objective
- Improvement in oxygen exchange
- Clearing of pulmonary edema as assessed by physical exam or chest x-ray
- Return of body weight to baseline level
- Stable serum biochemistry
- Absence of significant ventricular arrhythmias
- Absence of adverse effects of treatment
- ◆ Arrangements for follow-up
  - Medical appontment(s) booked
  - Home care nurse notified (496-1300)

For more information, please contact the Project Office 492-7427

APPENDIX C
CQIN Mission, Goals and Objectives

Mission
To improve patient outcomes through a shared vision, and implementation, of clinical quality improvement tools.

Goals
- To understand the scope and value of outcomes research
- To evaluate various options, such as clinical trials and critical pathways, for designing optimal clinical care

- To develop a perspective that integrates outcomes research with usual clinical practices and processes
- To embrace a perspective of health care that extends beyond secondary prevention and inpatient care to communities and healthier populations.

Objectives

- To conceive and develop appropriate research questions
- To design and execute studies to answer these questions in a feasible manner, with the highest degree of causal inference that can be reliably achieved
- To collect quality-assured data
- To analyze the data appropriately and propagate the results
- To attract funding to support the operations of the Network and dissemination of its research findings
- To foster communication and cooperation among health care practitioners, researchers, policy makers, and industry stakeholders in the health care system.

APPENDIX D

Representative CQIN Partnership/Governance Structure for the Project Entitled: Mortality risk and patterns of practice in 4,606 acute care patients with congestive heart failure. The relative importance of age, sex and medical therapy.

Source: The Clinical Quality Improvement Network (CQIN) Investigators.
(*Archives of Internal Medicine* (1996) 156: 1669–1673.)

Clinical Centres, Principal Investigators, and Coordinating Centre

University of Alberta Hospitals, Edmonton, AB: Koon Teo, PhD, Terrence Montague, MD, Margaret Ackman, PharmD, Marion Barnes, MSc, principal investigators; Colin Taylor, Graham Mansell, BMed.

Misericordia Hospital, Edmonton, AB: Paul Greenwood, MD, principal investigator; Anne Prosser, RN.
Royal Columbia Hospital, New Westminster, BC:, Ross Tsuyuki, PharmD, principal investigator; Carolyn Nilsson.

Surrey Memorial Hospital, Surrey, BC: Jan Kornder, MD, principal investigator.

Penticton Regional Hospital, Penticton, BC: Tom Ashton, MD, principal investigator.

Vernon Jubilee Hospital, Vernon, BC: Dan McLeod, MD, principal investigator.

St. Boniface Regional Hospital, Winnipeg, MB: Andrew Morris, MD, principal investigator; Kathy Robinson, RN.

Victoria General Hospital, Halifax, NS: David Johnstone, MD, principal investigator; Sharon Barnhill, RN, Pat Chatterton, BScN.

Project Office
Division of Cardiology, University of Alberta, Edmonton, AB: Terrence Montague, MD, Koon Teo, PhD, Marion Barnes, MSc, Margaret Ackman, PharmD, Patricia Montague, MSc, Glennora Dowding, Laurel Taylor, MBA, Sylvia Martin, RN, Drew Makinen, MD, Kyung Bay, PhD.

Coordinating Centre
Epidemiology Coordinating and Research (EPICORE) Centre, University of Alberta, Edmonton, AB: Koon Teo, PhD, Kyung Bay, PhD, Rita Yim, MHSA, Diane Cattelier, MSc, Joseph DeAlmeida, Terrence Montague, MD.

Writing Team
Margaret Ackman, PharmD, Patricia Montague, MSc, Koon Teo, PhD, Terrence Montague, MD.

APPENDIX E

Physician Order Sheet for Management of Patients with Heart Attack from a Representative CQIN Hospital, circa 1992–1996

Source: Reproduced, with permission, from *American Journal of Managed Care*

(The Clinical Quality Improvement Investigators 1998)

	☐ 6. **ASA:** 160 mg PO chew and swallow.
	If ASA **not** ordered, please state reason: _____ .
	☐ 7. **Beta blocker:**
	IV Beta blocker _____ , _____ mg followed by _____ mg po _____ .
	If Beta blocker **not** ordered, please state reason: _____ .
	8. **Thrombolytic:**
	☐ Trial thrombolytic as per _____ protocol.
	☐ **or** IV Streptokinase 1.5 million units as per Unit protocol
	☐ **or** IV t-PA 1.5-1.6 mg per kg as per Unit protocol
	If Thrombolytics **not** ordered, please state reason: _____ .

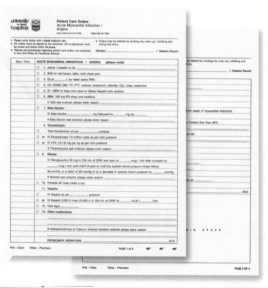

	☐ 13. **Other medications:**
	_____
	_____
	If Antidysrhythmics or Calcium channel blockers ordered please state reason:

APPENDIX F
ICONS Members and Affiliations
Regional Teams

Amherst

Highland View Regional Hospital
Drs. Gulshan Sawhney and Scott
Bowen (R)
Dr. Murray McCrossin (C)
Beth Munroe and Dawn Fage (P)
Cheryl Smith (RC)

Antigonish

St. Martha's Regional Hospital
Dr. Graham Miles (R)
Dr. Bill Booth (C)
Ian MacKeigan (P)
Maria DeCoste (RC)

Bridgewater

South Shore Regional Hospital
Dr. Ron Hatheway (R)
Dr. Ewart Morse (C)
Mike Laffin (P)
Marlene Wheatley (RC)

Dartmouth

Dartmouth General Hospital
Dr. Dale McMahon (R)
Heather Creighton (P)
Carol Atkinson (Data Quality
Coordinator)

Halifax

Queen Elizabeth II Health
    Sciences Centre
Dr. Iqbal Bata (R)
Dr. Kent Pottle (C)
Warren Meek (P)
Wilma Crowell (RC)

Kentville

Valley Regional Hospital
Dr. Michael O'Reilly (R)
Dr. Brian MacInnis (C)
Shelagh Campbell-Palmer (P)
Glenda O'Reilly (RC)

New Glasgow

Aberdeen Regional Hospital
Dr. Paul Seviour (R)
Dr. Colin Sutton (C)
Michelle MacDonald (P)
Kathy Saulnier (RC)

Sydney

Cape Breton Health Care Complex
Dr. Robert Baillie (R)
Dr. Paul Murphy (C)
John McNeil (P)
Mary MacNeil, Claudette Taylor (RC)

Truro

Colchester Regional Hospital
Dr. Masis Perk (R)
Dr. Michael Murray (C)
Bob MacDonald (P)
Dara Lee MacDonald (RC)

Yarmouth

Western Regional Health Centre
Dr. Rajender Parkash (R)
Dr. David Webster (C)
Jim MacLeod (P)
Kelly Goudey (RC)

R = Regional Leader; C = Primary Care Physician,
P = Pharmacist, RC = Research Coordinator

Executive:

Jafna Cox (Department of Medicine [Cardiology], Dalhousie
University; Project Officer); David Johnstone (Department of
Medicine [Cardiology], Dalhousie University; Project Chair);

Brenda Ryan (Nova Scotia Department of Health; Deputy Project Chair); Sarah Kramer (Nova Scotia Department of Health; Deputy Project Chair); Bonnie Cochrane, (Department of Patient Health, Merck Frosst Canada Ltd.; Deputy Project Officer); Joanna Nemis-White (Department of Patient Health, Merck Frosst Canada Ltd.; Deputy Project Officer).

Patients/Patient Representatives:
Robert Fitzner (Patient); Joan Fraser (Heart and Stroke Foundation of Nova Scotia); Yogi Joshi (Consumers' Association of Nova Scotia); Valerie White (Senior Citizens Secretariat).

Coordinating Centre:
Angela Mitchell-Lowery, Peter Hazelton (Manager of Operations); Jim Mathers (Data Analyst); Elizabeth Miguel (Administrative Assistant); Karl Roach, Lindsay Taylor and Tim Oben (Data Coordinators); Cindy Fiander, Brenda Preeper (Data Abstractors); Heather Merry (Veritas, Statistical Research Consulting, Halifax).

Dalhousie University:
Fred Burge, Wayne Putnam (Department of Family Medicine); Mike Allen (Continuing Medical Education); Gordon Flowerdew (Department of Community Health and Epidemiology); Ingrid Sketris (College of Pharmacy); Martin Gardner, Jonathan Howlett, Blair O'Neill and Malissa Wood (Cardiology); Greg Hirsch (Cardiac Surgery); David Anderson (Hematology).

QEII Health Sciences Centre:
Sandra Janes, Sandra Matheson and Karen MacRury-Sweet (Nursing); David Zitner (Quality Management).

Merck Frosst Canada Ltd.:
Gisèle Nakhlé, Kurt Ryan, Jeffery Sidel.

APPENDIX G
ICONS Care Map: Management of Anticoagulation in Atrial Fibrillation

Stable Patients: Dosing Algorithm to Achieve INR of 2.0 – 3.0

Warfarin Sodium: Monitoring and Dosage Adjustment in Stable Anticoagulated Patients (based on a starting dose of 4 mg/d)

INR	Action
> 10.0	Stop warfarin. Contact patient for examination.
7.0–10.0	Stop warfarin for 2 days; decrease weekly dosage by 25% or by 1 mg/d for next week (7 mg total); repeat PT in 1 week.
4.5–7.0	Decrease weekly dosage by 15% or by 1 mg/d for 5 days of next week (5 mg total); repeat PT in 1 week.
3.0–4.5	Decrease weekly dosage by 10% or by 1 mg/d for 3 days of next week (3 mg total); repeat PT in 1 week.
2.0–3.0	No change.
1.5–2.0	Increase weekly dosage by 10% or by 1 mg/d for 3 days of next week (3 mg total); repeat PT in 1 week.
< 1.5	Increase weekly dosage by 15% or by 1 mg/d for 5 days of next week (5 mg total); repeat PT in 1 week.

Modified from http://www.careinternet.com/caregiver/warfarin.htm
December 19, 2000.

Risk factors:
• Increasing age, a history of hypertension, prior TIA/stroke, impaired LV function, or diabetes compounds the risk of stroke.

Interfering factors:
• Ingestion of green, leafy vegetables and legumes, broccoli, asparagus, rhubarb etc. (in abundance) can decrease the effect of warfarin.
• Close attention is needed to INR when your patients are started on antibiotics, psychotropic drugs, corticosteroids, antiarrhythmics, anticonvulsants and certain other agents (see CPS).
• Alcohol consumption is not encouraged and should be *consumed only in moderation.*

The information on this card presents clinical guidelines as a supplement to, and not a substitute for, the expertise, skill, knowledge and judgement of health care practitioners in patient care, and is for guidance only.

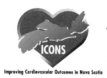

APPENDIX H

ICONS Care Map: Management of Heart Failure

Improving Cardiovascular Outcomes in Nova Scotia

Suspect Heart Failure
⇩
History/Physical Examination
↙
Exclude other possible
causes of signs/symptoms   ⇩

Heart Failure
⇩
Routine Tests (CBC, lytes, creatinine, Mg, chest X-ray, EKG)
⇩
Assess cardiac function (RNA / Echo + cath)
⇩
Treat underlying causes   ⇦ Determine Cause ⇨   Exclude causes that can
be treated with surgery

Predominant Systolic Dysfunction

⇩   ⇩   ⇩
Asymptomatic,   *Increasing signs/*   *CHF with preserved*
but EF<35–40%   *symptoms of failure*   *systolic function*
⇩   ⇩   ⇩
Treat with ACEi   Treat with ACEi   Individualize
Diuretic + salt restriction therapy, consult
Add beta-blocker   IM/Cardiology
Add digoxin

Add aldactone/spironolactone (FC III/IV)
Consider second vasodilator, e.g., AIIA
Assess for transplantation

Common Heart Failure Medication: Optimal Dose

ACE Inhibitors*:

Enalapril 10–20 mg bid (SOLVD)	Ramipril 5 mg bid (AIRE)
Lisinopril 35 mg od (ATLAS)	Captopril 50 mg tid (SAVE)

ß-blockers*:

Carvedilol 25 mg bid; 50 mg bid if > 180 lbs (COPERNICUS)	Bisoprolol 10 mg od (CIBIS II)	Metoprolol 100 mg bid† († Optimal dose not fully established—MERIT HF used long-acting formulation not available in Canada)

Digoxin 0.125 mg–0.25 mg od (DIG)
Spironolactone 25 mg od/bid (RALES)
Diuretic—minimum dose required to control congestive symptoms
* Start low, titrate to maximum tolerated/target dose.

Critical Path Guidelines

1. Usual Reasons for Hospital Admissions
▷ Non-adherence ▷ Volume overload ▷ Excessive Na intake
▷ Severe metabolic abnormalities ▷ Pulmonary/systemic embolus
▷ Acute myocardial ischemia/infarction ▷ Acute pulmonary edema
▷ Symptomatic cardiac rhythm disturbances ▷ Pneumonia/Bronchitis
▷ Intractable heart failure on maximal outpatient therapy ▷ Hypotension

2. Routine Monitoring and Investigations
▷ Daily Weights ▷ Blood pressure ▷ Heart Rate
▷ Chest X-ray ▷ 12-lead EKG ▷ Liver Function
▷ Risk factor assessment
▷ CBC, lytes, urea, creatinine, glucose, magnesium, TSH, Free T4
▷ Consult internal medicine/cardiology if not consulted < past 6 months

3. Special Diagnostic Tests (To assess cardiac ability and possible causes of heart failure)
▷ Echocardiogram ▷ Radionuclide angiogram (RNA)

4. Other Common Medications
▷ Angiotensin II Receptor Antagonists (AIIAs) ▷ Nitrates
▷ Lipid lowering/statins ▷ Potassium ▷ Magnesium
▷ Warfarin/aspirin/clopidogrel ▷ Avoid NSAIDS (incl. Cox2)

5. Components of Patient Education
▷ Sodium/fluid restriction ▷ Weight monitoring
▷ When/how to seek assistance ▷ Symptoms of decompensation

▷ Guidelines re: alcohol consumption ▷ Stress/Coping
▷ Diet and activity/exercise guidelines
▷ Medications and the importance of adherence

6. Criteria for Discharge from Acute Care

▷ Improvement of symptoms (orthopnea and/or PND)
▷ Improvement of O_2 exchange ▷ Stable serum biochemistry
▷ Education support in place ▷ Follow-up checklist
▷ Absence of adverse effects of treatment
▷ Discharge medications with plan to optimize
▷ Clearing of pulmonary edema, as assessed by physical exam and/or chest X-ray
▷ Return of body weight to baseline level (if good follow-up is in place, you can discharge before this occurs)

7. Arrangements for Follow-up

▷ Medical appointments arranged ▷ Home care in place

For more information, contact the ICONS Project Office at 902-473-7811.

APPENDIX I
ICONS Standardized Discharge Order Sheet

QE
Queen Elizabeth II
Health Sciences Centre

Cardiology Clinical Care Summary
Copies to: _____ _____
_____ _____

Admission Date (YYYY/MM/DD) ____02/09/26____   Discharge Date (YYYY/MM/DD): _____
Discharging Cardiologist: _____   Discharge/Transfer to: _____
Alternate level of care date: (Patient no longer requires acute care) (YYYY/MM/DD): _____
Most Responsible Diagnosis: ☐ Acute Myocardial Infarction - specify type and location _____
☐ Arrhythmia   ☐ Non Cardiac Chest Pain   ☐ Unstable Angina   ☐ Coronary Artery Disease
☐ Heart Failure   ☐ Other (Specify)_____
Comorbidities/Cardiac Risk Factors: ☐ Hypertension   ☐ Diabetes   ☐ Family History of IHD
☐ Smoking   ☐ Dyslipidemia   ☐ Obesity   ☐ Other (Specify) _____

Allergies (Specify) _____
Course in Hospital (include stress test, cardiac cath & procedure results)
_____
_____
_____
_____
_____
_____
_____

Pertinent Investigations / Lab Results
Peak CK _____ (U/L)   Total cholesterol _____ (MMOL/L)   LDL cholesterol _____ (MMOL/L)
EF _____ %   HDL cholesterol _____ (MMOL/L)   Triglycerides _____ (MMOL/L)
Other significant results:_____
Follow Up: ☐ Family Doctor _____   ☐ Cardiologist_____
☐ Heart Health Clinic   ☐ Diabetes Management Centre   ☐ Hypertension Clinic   ☐ Heart to Heart Program
☐ Cardiac Rehab   ☐ Stress Test   ☐ Echo   ☐ Other (Specify) _____
Recommendations for Family Doctor _____
_____
_____
_____

Medications on Discharge   (* unchanged from admission, ** altered, *** new)
1. _____   5. _____   9. _____
2. _____   6. _____   10. _____
3. _____   7. _____   11. _____
4. _____   8. _____   12. _____
Discharge Outcome Measures
Function: ☐ increased   ☐ unchanged   ☐ decreased   comment:_____
Comfort: ☐ increased   ☐ unchanged   ☐ decreased   comment:_____
Physician's Signature _____   Status _____
Print Name _____   Date (YYYY/MM/DD) _____
Discharging Cardiologist Signature _____   Date (YYYY/MM/DD) _____
Discharge Summary to follow ☐ yes   ☐ no   Dictated Date (YYYY/MM/DD) _____
Dictation Job # _____

QE7997 TR EXP. 00/09   White Copy - Health Records   Yellow Copy - Patient   Fax Referral

APPENDIX J
ICONS Provider Newsletter

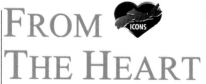

FROM THE HEART

Keeping in touch with ICONS

Visit our website at
www.icons.ns.ca

ICONS Project Participants' Newsletter

Volume 5, Number 2
Fall 2002

What's been happening with

FROM THE HEART

Keeping in touch with ICONS

Visit our website at
www.icons.ns.ca

ICONS Project Participants' Newsletter

Volume 6, Number 1
Winter 2003
Final Edition

u, the
of this

rts to
By
ituation
ell, to
va

What's been happening with ICONS

Current Size of the ICONS Registry (Oct 31, 2003)

- 68,074 hospital visits
- 37,659 individual patients
- 27,220 SF-36 surveys
- 31,682 interpreted ECGs
- 12,545 patients consented

The ICONS registry contains a large amount of information useful for improving the health of Nova Scotians.

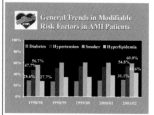

General Trends in Modifiable Risk Factors in AMI Patients

The above graph shows the increase of risk factors such as diabetes, high blood pressure, smoking and high cholesterol on the heart attack (AMI) population in Nova Scotia from 1998 – 2002.

The Role of Cardiac Enzymes in the Emergency Department

By Jim Scopie MT, RT

Emergency Department (ED) evaluation of patients with heart symptoms includes a blood test for cardiac enzyme testing. Cardiac enzymes are protein molecules released into the blood from heart muscle damaged due to a blocked artery.

People who come to the ED with heart symptom are assessed based on health history, physical examination, an electrocardiogram (ECG) and cardiac enzyme results. As the ECG is sometimes inconclusive, cardiac enzymes are used to determine if this event was actually a heart attack, an episode of angina or perhaps the symptoms are totally unrelated to the heart.

Cardiac enzymes most commonly used to assist in a patient's diagnosis are AST, LDH, CK, CK-MB and Troponin. These enzymes have a characteristic rise and fall pattern after a heart attack. A normal blood test upon arrival in the emergency room does not rule out a heart attack as it can often take 4 hours or more after symptoms first occur for the test to become abnormal and up to 24 hours for the enzyme to reach it's highest level. This is the reason that blood tests are often taken from the patient several times over a period of time. Eventually, enzyme levels in the blood return to normal.

To learn more about the cardiac enzymes mentioned above an excellent website to visit is www.labtestsonline.org.

more
/ou also
r the
ny
vince
sure:

nts my
to
uch as
r

respect.

APPENDIX K
ROCQ Project Outline

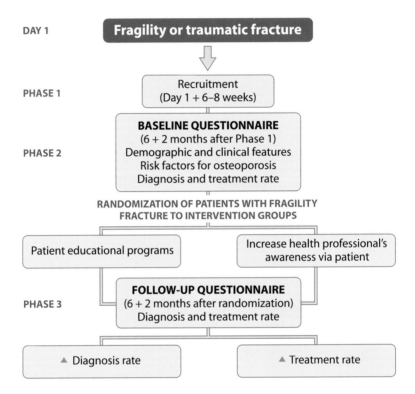

APPENDIX L
CURATA Treatment Algorithm for Osteoarthritis Patients

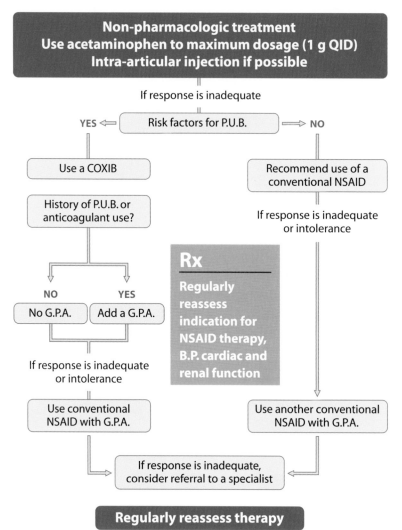

Non-pharmacologic treatment
Use acetaminophen to maximum dosage (1 g QID)
Intra-articular injection if possible

If response is inadequate

YES ⟸ Risk factors for P.U.B. ⟹ NO

Use a COXIB

Recommend use of a conventional NSAID

History of P.U.B. or anticoagulant use?

If response is inadequate or intolerance

Rx
Regularly reassess indication for NSAID therapy, B.P. cardiac and renal function

NO — No G.P.A.   YES — Add a G.P.A.

If response is inadequate or intolerance

Use conventional NSAID with G.P.A.

Use another conventional NSAID with G.P.A.

If response is inadequate, consider referral to a specialist

Regularly reassess therapy

G.P.A.: gastro-protective agent
P.U.B.: perforation, ulcer bleeding
B.P.: Blood pressure

APPENDIX M
Examples of Diabetes Hamilton Newsletters

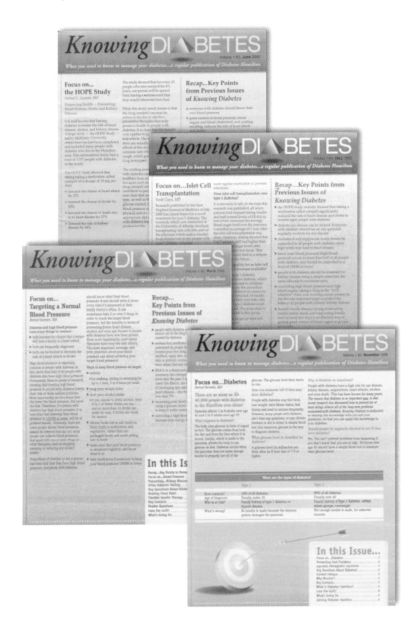

Bibliography

Ackman, M.L., J.B. Campbell, K.A. Buzak, R.T. Tsuyuki, T.J. Montague and K.K. Teo. 1999. "Use of Non-prescription Medications by Patients with Congestive Heart Failure." *Annals Pharmacotherapy* 33: 674–679.

Ackman, M.L., K.S. Harjee, G. Mansell, J.B. Campbell, K.K. Teo and T.J. Montague, for the Clinical Quality Improvement Network (CQIN) Investigators. 1996. "Cause-Specific Noncardiac Mortality in Patients with Congestive Heart Failure: A Contemporary Canadian Audit." *Canadian Journal of Cardiology* 12: 809–816.

Analysis Group/Economics. 2003. "The Value of Pharmaceuticals in Canada." http://www.canadapharma.org/ industry publications/valuemedicine.

Beaulieu, M., D. Choquette, E. Rahme, L. Bessette and R. Carrier. 2004. *In press.* "CURATA : A Patient Health Management Program for the Treatment of Osteoarthritis in Quebec: An Integrated Approach to Improving the Appropriate Use of Anti-inflammatory /Analgesic Medications." *American Journal of Managed Care.*

Boulet, L.-P., R.L. Thiverge, A. Amesse, F. Nunes, S. Francoeur and J.-P. Collet. 2002. "Towards Excellence in Asthma Management (TEAM): A Populational Disease-Management Model." *Journal of Asthma* 39: 341–350.

Butler, J., G. Khadim, K. Paul, S.F. Davis, W. Kronenberg, D.B. Chomsky, R.N. Pierson and J.R. Wilson. 2004. "Selection of Patients for Heart Transplantation in the Current Era of Heart

Failure Therapy." *Journal of the American College of Cardiology* 43: 787–793.

Butler, C., S. Rollnick and N. Stott. 1996. "The Practitioner, the Patient and Resistance to Change: Recent Ideas on Compliance." *Canadian Medical Association Journal* 154: 1357–1362.

Canadian Cardiovascular Collaboration, The. 1995. "Collaborative Cardiovasular Clinical Trials in Canada." *Canadian Journal of Cardiology* 11: 649–657.

Clark, R. 1971. *Einstein: The Life and Times*. New York: World Publishing Company.

Clinical Quality Improvement Network (CQIN) Investigators, The. 1995. "Low Incidence of Assessment and Modification of Risk Factors in Acute Care Patients at High Risk for Cardio-vascular Events, Particularly among Females and the Elderly." *American Journal of Cardiology* 76: 570–573.

_____. 1996. "Mortality Risk and Patterns of Practice in 4,606 Acute Care Patients with Congestive Heart Failure: The Relative Importance of Age, Sex and Medical Therapy." *Archives of Internal Medicine* 156: 1669–1673.

_____. 1998. "Influence of a Critical Path Management Tool in the Treatment of Acute Myocardial Infarction." *American Journal of Managed Care* 4: 1243–1251.

Cox, J.L., on behalf of the ICONS Investigators. 1999. "Optimizing Disease Management at a Health Care System Level: The Improving Cardiovascular Outcomes in Nova Scotia (ICONS) Study." *Canadian Journal of Cardiology* 15: 787–796.

Cutler, D., and M. McClellan. 2001. "Is Technological Change in Medicine Worth It?" *Health Affairs* 20: 11–29.

Digitalis Investigation Group, The. 1996. "Rationale, Design, Implementation and Baseline Characteristics of Patients in the DIG Trial: A Large, Simple Trial to Evaluate the Effect of Digitalis on Mortality in Heart Failure." *Controlled Clinical Trials* 17: 77–97.

_____. 1997. "The Effect of Digoxin on Mortality and Morbidity in Patients with Heart Failure." *New England Journal of Medicine* 336: 525–533.

Disease Management Association of America 2004. "Definition of Disease Management." http://www.dmaa.org/definition.html.

Epstein, R.E., and L.M. Sherwood. 1996. "From Outcomes Research to Disease Management: A Guide for the Perplexed." *Annals of Internal Medicine* 124: 832–837.

Glover, J.A. "The Incidence of Tonsillectomy in School Children." *Proceedings of the Royal Society of Medicine* 1938; 31: 1219-1236.

Gross, D. 2004. "Whose Problem Is Health Care?" *The New York Times* (February 8): BU 6.

Heart Outcomes Prevention Evaluation Study Investigators, The. 2000. "Effects of an Angiotensin-Converting-Enzyme Inhibitor, Ramipril, on Death from Cardiovascular Causes, Myocardial Infarction, and Stroke in High-Risk Patients." *New England Journal of Medicine* 342: 145–153.

HOPE Study Investigators, The. 1996. "The HOPE (Heart Outcomes Prevention Evaluation) Study: The Design of a Large Simple Randomized Trial of an Angiotensin-Converting Enzyme Inhibitor (Ramipril) and Vitamin E in Patients at High Risk of Cardiovascular Events." *Canadian Journal of Cardiology* 12: 127–137.

Horn, S.D., P.D. Sharkey and J. Gassaway. 1996. "Managed Care Outcomes Project: Study Design, Baseline Patient Characteristics, and Outcome Measures." *American Journal of Managed Care* 2: 237–247.

Laurier, C., Blais, L., Kennedy, W., Koné, A., Pare, M., Perron, M., Pitre, P. Surveillance épidémiologique de l'asthme au Québec et variations régionales, 1999–2001: une analyse des banques de données. Faculté de Pharmacie et Faculté de Médecine, Université de Montréal, et Department de Géographie, Université de Québec a Montréal, Juin 2004.

Lichtenberg, F.R. 1998. "Pharmaceutical Innovation, Mortality Reduction, and Economic Growth." National Bureau of Economic Research Working Paper # 6569. May 1998: 1–30.

_____. 2004. "The Impact of New Drug Launches on Longevity: Evidence from Longitudinal Disease-Level Data from 52 Countries, 1982–2001." *National Bureau of Economic Research*, Working Paper w9754. http://papers.nber.org/papers/mail/w9754.

Marinker, M., ed. 1997. *From Compliance to Concordance: Achieving Shared Goals in Medicine Taking*. London: Royal Pharmaceutical Society; Merck, Sharp and Dohme.

McAlister, F.A., L. Taylor, K. Teo, R.T. Tsuyuki, M.L. Ackman, R. Yim and T.J. Montague, for the Clinical Quality Improvement Network Investigators. 1999. "The Treatment and Prevention of Coronary Heart Disease in Canada: Do Older Patients Receive Efficacious Therapies?" *Journal of the American Geriatric Society* 47 (1): 911–918.

McAlister, F.A., K. Teo, M. Taher, T.J. Montague, D. Humen, L. Cheung, M. Kiaii and P.W. Armstrong. 1999. "Insights into the Contemporary Epidemiology and Outpatient Management of Congestive Heart Failure." *American Heart Journal* 138: 87–94.

Mitnitski, A.B., A.J. Mogilner, X. Song, J.L. Cox and K. Rockwood. 2003. "A Score for Predicting of the Risk of Death Following Acute Myocardial Infarction." *Circulation* 108 (17): IV–714.

Montague, T. 2003a. "Outcomes in Health Care: Motivation, Measures and Drivers at the Population Level." in *Emotional & Interpersonal Dimensions of Health Services: Enriching the Art and Science of Care*, edited by L. Dube, G. Ferland and D.S. Moskowitz, 151–161. Montreal-Kingston-London-Ithaca: McGill-Queen's University Press.

Montague, T. 2003b. "What Determines Health and Quality of Life? Health as Good Economics." *Association of Canadian Medical Colleges Forum* 33: 12–14.

Montague, T., M. Barnes, L. Taylor, A. Ignaszewski, D. Modry, R. Wensel, D. Humen and K. Teo. 1996. "Assessing Appropriateness of Treatment: A Case Study of Transplantation in Congestive Heart Failure." *Canadian Journal of Cardiology* 12: 47–52.

Montague, T., and S. Cavanaugh. 2004. "Seeking Value in Pharmaceutical Care: Balancing Quality, Access and Efficiency." Healthcare*Papers* 4: 51–58.

Montague, T., J. Cox, S. Kramer, J. Nemis-White, B. Cochrane, M. Wheatley, Y. Joshi, R. Carrier, J.-P. Gregoire and D. Johnstone, for the ICONS Investigators. 2003. "Improving Cardiovascular Outcomes in Nova Scotia: ICONS, a Successful Public/Private Partnership in Primary Health Care." *Hospital Quarterly* 6: 32–38.

Montague, T., P. Montague, M. Barnes, L. Taylor, L. Wowk, K. Fassbender, M. Ackman, S. Martin and K. Teo, for the Clinical Quality Improvement Network (CQIN) Investigators. 1996. "Acute Myocardial Infarction in Canada: New Epidemiologic Insights on Incidence, Therapy and Risk." *Journal of Thrombosis and Thrombolysis* 3: 101–105.

Montague, T., J. Sidel, B. Erhardt, G. Nakhle, L. Caron, D. Croteau, M. Kader, J. Haket, K. Skilton and B. McLeod. 1997. "Patient Health Management: A Promising Paradigm in Canadian Healthcare." *American Journal of Managed Care* 3: 1175–1182.

Montague, T., L. Taylor, M. Barnes, M. Ackman, R. Tsuyuki, R. Wensel, R. Williams, D. Catellier and K. Teo, for the Clinical Quality Improvement Network (CQIN) Investigators. 1995. "Can Practice Patterns Be Successfully Altered? Examples from Cardiovascular Medicine." *Canadian Journal of Cardiology* 11: 487–492.

Montague, T., K. Teo, L. Taylor, F. McAlister, M. Ackman and R. Tsuyuki, for the Investigators and Staff of the Heart Function Clinic, University of Alberta Hospitals, and the Clinical Quality Improvement Network (CQIN). 1998. in "In Pursuit of Optimal Care and Outcomes for Patients with Congestive Heart Failure: Insights from the Past Decade." *Angiotensin II Receptor Blockade: Physiological and Clinical Implications*, edited by N.S. Dhalla, P. Zahradka, I.M.C. Dixon and R.E. Beamish, 221–232. Boston: Kluwer Academic Publishers.

Montague, T., R. Tsuyuki and K. Teo. 1998. "Improving Women's Health Quality: The Value of Closing the Care Gap." *Hospital Quarterly* 2: 36–39.

243

Montague, T., R. Wong, R. Crowell, K. Bay, D. Marshall, W. Tymchak, K. Teo and N. Davies. 1990. "Acute Myocardial Infarction: Contemporary Risk and Management in Older versus Younger Patients." *Canadian Journal of Cardiology* 6: 241–246.

Nordhaus, W.D. 2002. "The Health of Nations: Irving Fisher and the Contribution of Improved Longevity to Living Standard." National Bureau of Economic Research Working Paper # 8818, February 2002: 1–61.

Osler, W. 1910. "The Faith That Heals." *The British Medical Journal* 1: 1470–1472.

Rosenstock, I.M. 1974. "Historical Origins of the Health Belief Model." *Health Education Monograms* 2 (4): 328–335.

Schlansky, S.J., A.R. Levy. 2002. "Effect of Number of Medications on Cardiovascular Therapy Adherence." *Annals of Pharmacotherapy* 36: 1532–1539.

Sharpe, H.M., D.D. Sin, E. Andrews, R.L. Cowie and S.F.P. Man. In press. "Alberta Strategy to Help Manage Asthma (ASTHMA): A Provincial Initiative to Improve Outcomes for Individuals with Asthma." Healthcare*Papers*.

Sidel, J., K. Ryan and J. Nemis-White. 1998. "Shaping the Healthcare Environment through Evidence-Based Medicine." *Hospital Quarterly* 2: 29–33.

Smith D. 2004. "At Ease with a Pen, but Also with a Stethoscope." *The New York Times* (March 16): D5.

SOLVD Investigators, The. 1990. "Studies of Left Ventricular Dysfunction (SOLVD): Rationale, Design and Methods: Two Trials That Evaluate the Effect of Enalapril in Patients with Reduced Ejection Fraction." *American Journal of Cardiology* 66: 315–322.

_____. 1991. "Effect of Enalapril on Survival in Patients with Reduced Left Ventricular Ejection Fractions and Congestive Heart Failure." *New England Journal of Medicine* 325: 293–302.

_____. 1992. "Effect of Enalapril on Mortality and the Development of Heart Failure in Asymptomatic Patients with Reduced Left Ventricular Ejection Fractions." *New England Journal of Medicine* 327: 685–691.

Taylor, L.K. 2001. *Contemporary Physician Practice Patterns: Insights from Institutional Theory.* Edmonton: University of Alberta Press.

Teo, K., J. Burton, C. Buller, S. Plante, D. Catellier, W. Tymchak, V. Dzavik, D. Taylor, S. Yokoyama and T. Montague, on behalf of the SCAT Investigators. 2000. "Long-Term Effects of Cholesterol Lowering and Angiotensin-Converting Enzyme Inhibition on Coronary Atherosclerosis: The Simvastatin/Enalapril Coronary Atherosclerosis Trial (SCAT)." *Circulation* 102: 1748–1754.

Teo, K.K., J.R. Burton, C. Buller, S. Plante, S. Yokoyama and T.J. Montague, on behalf of the SCAT Investigators. 1997. "Rationale and Design Features of a Clinical Trial Examining the Effects of Cholesterol Lowering and Angiotensin Converting Enzyme Inhibition on Coronary Atherosclerosis." *Canadian Journal of Cardiology* 13: 591–599.

Teo, K., J. Burton, J. DeAmeida, S. Dolezar, P. Montague, V. Dzavik, W. Tymchak, D. Taylor and T. Montague, for the Simvastatin /Enalapril Coronary Atherosclerosis Trial (SCAT) Investigators. 1997. "Quantitative Relation of Electrocardiographic and Angiocardiographic Measures of Risk in Patients with Coronary Atherosclerosis." *Canadian Journal of Cardiology* 13: 363–369.

Tsuyuki, R., J. Johnson, K. Teo, S. Simpson, M. Ackman, R. Biggs, A. Cave, W.C. Chang, V. Dzavik, K. Farris, D. Galvin, W. Semchuk, J. Taylor, for the Study of Cardiovacular Risk Intervention by Pharmacists (SCRIP) Investigators. 2002. "A Randomized Trial of the Effect of Community Pharmacist on Cholesterol Risk Management: The Study of Cardiovascular Risk Intervention by Pharmacists (SCRIP)." *Archives of Internal Medicine* 162: 1149–1155.

Tsuyuki, R., K. Olson, A. Dubyk, T. Schindel and J. Johnson. 2004. "Effect of Community Pharmacist Intervention on Cholesterol Levels in Patients at High Risk of Cardiovascular Events: The Second Study of Cardiovascular Risk Intervention by Pharmacists (SCRIP-plus)." *American Journal of Medicine* 116: 130–133.

Tsuyuki, R., D. Sin, H. Sharpe, R. Cowie and P. Man, for the Alberta Strategy to Help Manage Asthma (ASTHMA) Investigators. 2004. *submitted.* "Management of Asthma among Community-Based Primary Care Physicians." *Chest.*

Tsuyuki, R.T., K.K. Teo, R.M. Ikuta, K.S. Bay, P.V. Greenwood and T.J. Montague. 1994. "Mortality Risk and Patterns of Practice in 2070 Patients with Acute Myocardial Infarction 1987–92: The Relative Importance of Age, Sex and Medical Therapy." *Chest* 105: 1687–1692.

Tugwell, P., K.J. Bennett, D.L. Sackett and R.B. Haynes. 1985. "The Measurement Iterative Loop: A Framework for the Critical Appraisal of Need, Benefits, and Costs, of Health Interventions." *Journal of Chronic Diseases* 38: 339–351.

Wahl, C., J.-P. Gregoire, K.K. Teo, M. Beaulieu, S.. Labelle, B. Leduc, B. Cochrane, L. Lapointe and T. Montague. 2004. *In Press.* "Concordance, Compliance and Adherence in Health Care: Closing Gaps and Improving Outcomes." *Healthcare Quarterly.*

White, K.L. 1993. "Health Care Research: Old Wine in New Bottles." *The Pharos* 56: 12–16.

Index

evolution of, 4–6

increased spending to close, 203

measurement of, 43–46. 44f, 45f, 46f

multiple stakeholders, role of, 53–54

older patients. *See* older patients care gap

overlapping responsibilities for, 41

poor compliance. *See* compliance gap

popularity of term, 35

prediction of, 38–39

suboptimal diagnosis of patients at risk, 41–42

suboptimal prescribing of efficacious therapies. *See* prescribing gap

case management, 15

Catellier, Diane, 118

cause-and effect attribution hierarchy, 104

Centre for Community Pharmacy Research and Interdisciplinary Strategies (COMPRIS), 122

chronological age, *vs.* biological age, 91–92

Clinical Quality Improvement Network (CQIN)

see also patient health management (PHM)

best treatment intentions, 210

community-based partnerships, 100

described, 137–141

EPICORE support, 120

measurement and feedback processes, 100

mission, goals and objectives, 224–225

physician order sheet, 227

proven therapies, and survival rates, 37f

representative partnership/governance structure, 225–226

clinical trials

see also outcomes research; randomized clinical trials

Hawthorne Effect, power of, 124

increased knowledge of best care, 37

incremental benefit of new therapies, 36

as measurement, 5

real-world effectiveness, comparison with, 37–38

clinicians

medical practice, context of, 30

patient-provider relationship. *See* patient-provider relationship

shortage of, 30–31

College of Physicians, 169

Columbia's Graduate School of Business, 74

combining, 194–195

commitment, 191–192

communication

components of, 193

of important system parameters, 215

patient-doctor communication, and compliance gap, 58, 62

patient-physician communication, value of, 134–135